skinny-
size it

Also by Molly Morgan

The Skinny Rules

skinny-size it

101 RECIPES
THAT WILL FILL YOU UP AND SLIM YOU DOWN

MOLLY MORGAN, RD, CDN, CSSD

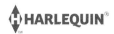

Skinny-Size It
ISBN-13: 978-0-373-89298-3
© 2014 by Molly Morgan, RD, CDN, CSSD

The health advice presented in this book is intended only as an informative resource guide to help you make informed decisions; it is not meant to replace the advice of a physician or to serve as a guide to self-treatment. Always seek competent medical help for any health condition or if there is any question about the appropriateness of a procedure or health recommendation.

Library of Congress Cataloging-in-Publication Data on file with the publisher.

www.Harlequin.com

Printed in U.S.A.

Contents

To my husband and our two little guys,
the best supporters.

Acknowledgments

Thank you, thank you, thank you to my husband and our two little guys, who happily tried every recipe in this book because for each recipe that turns out great, there are definitely some that flop in between! Our friends and family are so supportive and have also been taste testers throughout this process and I'm forever grateful for their recipe inspiration, input and suggestions!

Lastly, this book would not be a reality without Holly Schmidt from Hollan Publishing or my Harlequin editor, Sarah Pelz. Your ongoing support and encouragement is incredible and made my second Skinny book come to life!

Introduction

Life has gotten so busy that for many people, meals are primarily purchased and consumed at restaurants and drive-throughs or feature premade foods taken out of bags and boxes at home. Meals eaten out at restaurants are typically higher in fat, including saturated fat, sodium and sugar as compared to what you would make at home. Sometimes restaurant dishes seem like a healthy choice, yet when they arrive at the table, you find that they are swimming in a pool of melted butter or are loaded with salt.

Preparing and eating meals at home gives you control over the quality of the foods you consume and the quantity of fat, sugar and salt added. In addition, when you cook, you burn calories: approximately thirty minutes of cooking translates into ninety calories burned, and the cleanup burns another fifty calories, for a total of 140 calories burned (based on a 150-pound person). By preparing just three meals per week and doing the cleanup, you could burn 21,840 calories a year, which equals six pounds' worth of calories. And if you prepared *Skinny-Size It* recipes—creating healthier alternatives by skipping and swapping out high-fat, high-calorie ingredients and avoiding certain cooking methods—you would consume fewer calories.

After writing *The Skinny Rules,* I was so excited to write *Skinny-Size It,* because eating healthy can taste great and you can make meals that fill your plate! This book is not about cutting down portion sizes to keep calories in check. Rather the recipes in *Skinny-Size It* call for plenty of fruits, vegetables, whole grains, beans and spices to maximize portion sizes while focusing on flavor from aromatic vegetables, herbs and spices, allowing you to enjoy a full plate of food for a much lower calorie price tag. I am always on the lookout for recipe ideas: I snap pictures of dishes I find appealing, and I read recipes in cooking magazines. Then I head to the grocery store for the ingredients, return to our kitchen and re-create the recipes in a way that makes them as healthy as can be.

You may notice there are a lot of vegetarian and vegan recipes throughout this book. While I have always worked a lot of fruits, vegetables, whole grains, nuts and seeds into my eating routine, for over a year I have gone mostly meatless and have limited the amount of processed foods, high-fat dairy foods and eggs in my eating routine. Why did I revise my eating plan in this way? Research has proven the health benefits of a plant-based diet: weigh less and have a reduced risk for certain types of cancer, heart disease and diabetes. In general, Americans overdo protein and animal foods, consuming too much. Have you ever stopped to consider that nearly every dish on most restaurant menus (and perhaps even your own home dishes) contains either meat, eggs, cheese or other dairy products, and some even feature a combination of all four? Never eating meat, eggs, cheese or other dairy products may not be right for you. However, eating more minimally processed fruits, vegetables, whole grains, nuts and seeds would certainly be beneficial for everyone, since most people do not eat enough of these foods. Every recipe in *Skinny-Size It* incorporates them.

Perhaps you were wondering why there are no dessert recipes in this book. The reason I decided to exclude dessert recipes is that while removing a few grams of fat or adding a bit of fiber to a dessert recipe certainly would "health it up," at the end of the day, it would still be a dessert. I figured that my energy was best spent on developing recipes that could serve as more of a foundation for eating routines, rather than just as icing on the cake. If you're really craving something sweet at the end of your meals, this book offers a few delicious and satisfying options, such as Baked Apple Pie Parfaits and Apple Cinnamon Chia Swirl Pudding, both in the Snacks and Appetizers chapter.

It is always important to keep the bottom line in mind when it comes to meals: food is fuel. Would you put a type of gas in your car that would stop it from working efficiently? Probably not. Think of foods as fuel for your body, and consider that the right mix certainly can help you to feel and look your best. Last but not least, incorporating the fresh flavors of fruits, vegetables, whole grains, nuts and seeds, and spices and herbs can make healthy recipes taste great. So with that in mind, what are you going to cook today?

STOCKING YOUR SKINNY KITCHEN

Having a supply of certain ingredients and tools on hand makes it much easier to pull together Skinny meals. Check your cupboards to see which of the ingredients listed here you keep on hand and which ones you need to add to your shopping list.

Fresh herbs and spices

Fresh herbs, like dill and parsley, are too delicate to stock up on in large quantities. On the other hand, fresh gingerroot, a spice that is a necessity when it comes to Skinny cooking, is hearty and holds up well when stored in the refrigerator. If you like having plants, try keeping potted herbs that you use routinely in cooking, such as basil, mint, oregano, parsley and rosemary. I like to keep at least one fresh herb (a favorite is rosemary) plant growing in our kitchen year round, and seasonally we grow the other herbs in the garden. I have to say that herbs are relatively simple to grow. Two that I especially like to keep on hand during the summer months are mint and basil.

Aromatic vegetables

The foundation of flavor in many *Skinny-Size It* recipes comes from aromatic vegetables including garlic, onions, peppers and celery. These vegetables are full of flavor and deliver vitamins and minerals like vitamin C, folate, manganese, potassium and vitamin A. Consider aromatic vegetables like these staples of Skinny cooking!

Vinegars

To add great flavor to sauces and dressings, keep a variety of vinegars in your pantry, including balsamic vinegar, white balsamic vinegar, red wine vinegar, white wine vinegar and rice vinegar.

Oils

The quality of oil varies, and you definitely get what you pay for. For example, extra-virgin olive oil is more expensive than other olive oil versions because it comes from the first press of the olives and is the most nutrient rich and has a rich olive flavor! In comparison, light olive oil is a more processed oil that is lighter in flavor (but has the same amount of calories and fat). In addition, oils have different smoke points (the maximum temperature to which they can be heated before they break down) and flavor profiles.

The best oils for baking, oven cooking and stir-frying are canola oil, grapeseed oil, extra-virgin olive oil and peanut oil. The best oils for light sautéing, for making sauces and for cooking over low heat are sesame oil, sunflower oil, walnut oil and coconut oil. Keep on hand oils that are suitable for all these tasks. If I were to pick my top two favorite oils, they would be extra-virgin olive oil and sesame oil.

Specialty oils, such as fish oil and flaxseed oil, offer health benefits but do not hold up well when used with heat, so stick to adding these only to smoothies and/or drizzling on a finished recipe. When it comes to these oils, if some is good, more is not better. In large doses (over three grams per day), both fish oil and flaxseed oil can have a thinning effect on the blood and can cause bruising, nosebleeds, nausea and other health issues.

Meat substitutes

There are two meat substitutes that are Skinny staples: tofu and tempeh. Several varieties of tofu are commonly available, including:

- **Silken tofu:** has a soft texture and a high water content, and is excellent in smoothies and dips and as a swap for eggs.
- **Firm tofu:** has been slightly pressed but still retains some water, and is perfect for stir-frying and sautéing.
- **Extra-firm tofu:** is well pressed and has less water, and thus is suitable for marinating and grilling.

Tempeh is made through a natural fermentation process that binds soybeans, and this fermentation process results in a higher protein, fiber and vitamin content. Four ounces of tempeh contains twenty-two grams of protein and twelve grams of fiber. The firm texture of tempeh makes it excellent for marinating and using on sandwiches.

Dairy and eggs

Many foods from the dairy aisle, like plain nonfat Greek yogurt and light cheddar cheese, are essential Skinny ingredients, and once you start working them into your recipes, you won't turn back. Generally, when it comes to dairy foods, such as yogurt, cheese, cream cheese and cottage cheese, always select low-fat (1 percent) or light products. Typically, I do not suggest fat-free dairy products, because they often don't melt or perform as well in recipes. One exception to that rule, however, is plain nonfat Greek yogurt. Because of the way Greek yogurt is made, the nonfat version holds up well in recipes and you almost don't realize that the fat isn't there.

When it comes to eggs, paying extra for omega-3 eggs is worth it, as these eggs provide a boost of heart-helping omega-3 fats.

Butter or margarine? Both are high in total fat: butter is high in saturated fat, while margarine, which is made with vegetable oils, is lower in saturated fat. It really comes down to your personal flavor preference. Since both are high in fat, a limited amount of either should be consumed. If you do choose margarine, make certain to choose a brand that meets two criteria: it has zero grams of trans fat *and* it does not have partially hydrogenated oil, a trans fat, listed on the food label. This is important because food-labeling laws allow companies to declare on the Nutrition Facts panel that foods with less than half a gram of trans fat have zero grams. To be certain that a particular food really has zero grams of trans fat, you should review the ingredient list, looking for the words "partially hydrogenated oil." If the words "partially hydrogenated oil" are listed, this means trans fat and although a food may contain less than half a gram of trans fat per serving, over time that amount adds up, and the goal is to avoid trans fat completely because of its negative impact on heart health.

Flavor boosters

There are ingredients, such as dried herbs and spices, that add great flavor to recipes, and you will want to keep these in your Skinny cupboard. Having a variety of dried herbs and spices on hand is a must. These include dried basil, celery seed, cilantro, cinnamon, cumin, dry mustard, ginger, garlic powder, onion powder, oregano, parsley, paprika, black pepper and white pepper. If you make a *Skinny-Size It* recipe or one of your own that you feel needs more flavor, before you reach for the salt shaker, try adding an herb or a spice, as it will boost the flavor without adding sodium.

Table salt or sea salt? The biggest difference between table salt and sea salt is in how they are processed. Table salt is mined from salt deposits and then processed, while sea salt is made by evaporating ocean water and usually not processed. Both have the same amount of sodium by weight, which keeps the playing field level. When it comes to adding some salt to a recipe, my personal preference is to add sea salt because the coarser texture packs a bigger sodium taste and can result in less overall salt added for the same taste impact.

A word on sodium: A majority of sodium intake comes from processed foods; in fact, about 75 percent of sodium comes from processed foods or from the salt added to foods in restaurants and other food service locations. Basically, all Americans consume more sodium than they need, with an average intake of about 3,400 milligrams per day. The goal for healthy adults is to consume 2,300 milligrams or less sodium per day. The goal for adults who have high blood pressure, chronic kidney disease or diabetes, and for those who are African American, is to have 1,500 milligrams or less sodium per day. Note: if you are very active for more than one to two hours per day, your sodium needs may be higher because of your rate of sweating. All the recipes in *Skinny-Size It* skip salt or skimp on the amount of added salt to keep the overall sodium content low. Another key is adding the salt to a dish just before serving, which keeps the salty taste at the top of the dish, instead of dispersing it throughout the dish when it is added during cooking.

Other flavor boosters to keep on hand that are healthier alternatives include lite soy sauce, light coconut milk, low-sodium broth and liquid smoke.

Nuts, seeds and dried fruit

Some *Skinny-Size It* recipes contain nuts and seeds, which provide healthy (unsaturated) fats and crunch, as well as dried fruit, which lends sweetness. These include walnuts, almonds, raw cashews, sunflower seeds, ground flaxseed, chia seeds, dried cranberries, dried apricots, dried mango and raisins.

The nuts, seeds and dried fruit you include in a recipe is up to you, so keep on hand those you like best.

The sweet stuff

Skinny-Size It recipes skimp on the amount of sugar added. Making salad dressings and sweet sauces, such as barbecue sauce, from scratch allows you to control the quantity of sugar added. It is a good idea to keep a mix of sweeteners on hand and to select the one that works best in each recipe. Sweeteners include granulated sugar, pure maple syrup, agave nectar, honey and brown sugar.

Is agave nectar a health food? Agave nectar is a mix of fructose (90 percent) and glucose (10 percent), though the amounts of each vary based on how the sugar is processed. Agave nectar is produced from *aguamiel,* that is, the sap of the agave plant, and is processed until it reaches more or less the consistency of maple syrup. It has a very light taste, and one of its perks is that it is about one and a half times sweeter than table sugar. However, it also has more calories compared to table sugar: sixty calories per tablespoon versus forty calories per tablespoon for sugar. So while agave nectar is used in some of the *Skinny-Size It* recipes to avoid adding table sugar, it should still be used in moderation.

Grains

The recommendation set forth in the USDA's *Dietary Guidelines for Americans* (2010) is to make at least half your grains whole grains. The *Skinny-Size It* goal is to make almost all your grains whole grains, as they not only are more nutrient rich than their stripped-down counterparts, but also add excellent flavor and texture to recipes. Whole grains and whole-grain products to stock up on include brown rice, steel-cut oats, rolled oats (also called old-fashioned oats), quinoa (red, white, black/purple), whole-wheat panko bread crumbs, oat flour, whole-wheat flour, white whole-wheat flour, whole-wheat pasta, soba (100 percent buckwheat) noodles, wheat bran, cornmeal and buckwheat flour.

SKINNY TOOLS

Having the right mix of ingredients is a must, and having the essential tools to prepare healthy foods can make the job easier and, in some cases, more enjoyable too! Check out the list of Skinny tools to have on hand. If your kitchen is missing some of these tools, add them to your wish list and slowly work on getting them.

- Garlic press—e.g., OXO Garlic Press, approximately $20.00
- Salad dressing shaker—e.g., Tupperware Quick Shake Container, $15.00–$20.00
- Mini food processor (1½-cup)—e.g., Black & Decker 1½-Cup Food Chopper, $13.00–$20.00
- Large food processor (5- to 9-cup)—e.g., Cuisinart 5-Cup Food Processor, $270.00
- Cast iron skillet (12-inch)—e.g., Lodge Cast Iron Skillet, $18.00
- Large stainless-steel skillet (14-inch)— e.g., All-Clad, $180.00–$200.00
- Stockpots and soup pots (small [3-quart], medium [5-quart] and large [8+-quart])—prices vary
- Blender and/or immersion blender— e.g., Bamix Immersion Blender, $179.00

- Cut-resistant gloves—e.g., Microplane Cut-Resistant Gloves, $15.00
- Salad spinner—e.g., OXO Salad Spinner (small or large), $24.00–$30.00
- Mini colander (2- to 3-cup)—e.g., Crate and Barrel, $7.00
- Wok (13-inch)—e.g., Calphalon Stainless Wok, $100.00
- Rice cooker (works great for quinoa too!)—e.g., Oster Rice Cooker and Food Steamer, $20.00
- Pizza stone—e.g., Breville Smart Oven Pizza Stone, $30.00

SKINNY SKIMPS, SWAPS AND SKIPS

The *Skinny-Size It* recipes have already made these skimps, swaps and skips for you! You can use this chart to move some of your not so Skinny recipes over to the Skinny side.

Whole eggs

- **Swap one whole egg** for two egg whites. This works great in baking. For every whole egg you swap out, you will save 184 milligrams of cholesterol and five grams of fat.
- **Swap one whole egg** for two ounces of silken tofu. This works great in egg scrambles.
- **Use an egg replacer** (such as Ener-G Egg Replacer) made with potato and tapioca flours in baked goods to forgo eggs altogether. Note that 1½ teaspoons

egg replacer + 2 tablespoons warm water equals one egg. Works great in cookies, quick breads, muffins and brownies.

Flour

- **Replace at least half the non-whole-grain flour** in most recipes with 100 percent whole-grain flour (whole wheat, white whole wheat or buckwheat). This works especially great with cookies, muffins and quick breads.
- **Swap one-quarter of the flour** in a recipe for flaxseed meal to boost the fiber content of a recipe.

Milk

- **Swap low-fat cow's milk** for almond milk and save sixty calories per cup and gain 1½ grams of monounsaturated fat per cup (from the almonds)!
- **Swap whole milk or 2 percent milk** for 1 percent milk or skim milk to reduce the calories and fat in a recipe.
- **Swap buttermilk** for the same amount of low-fat milk plus one tablespoon of vinegar.
- **Swap heavy cream** for cashew cream, which is loaded with heart-healthy unsaturated fat instead of saturated fat. Soak one cup of raw cashews overnight (or for at least thirty minutes), drain most of the water, reserving it, and blend the cashews in a blender until creamy, adding a teaspoon of the

reserved water at a time, if needed. Stir the cashew cream into soups and sauces to thicken them!

Oil

- **Reduce the amount of oil** in a recipe by half or skip it all together (depending on the recipe).
- **For baked items,** such as muffins and quick breads, substitute equal parts unsweetened applesauce for oil.
- **Sauté vegetables without any oil!** Each tablespoon of oil, even extra-virgin olive oil, adds 120 calories and fourteen grams of fat to a dish. Even though it is healthy fat, it still has calories, and it is easy to overdo it.

Sweet onions

When making soups and sauces, start with sautéed sweet onions to add fresh flavor and to limit the amount of heavier ingredients that must be added during cooking.

Sugar

Skimp on or skip the added sugar in recipes and rely on the flavors of the ingredients instead. Typically, at least a third of the sugar in a recipe can be removed without altering the texture of the finished product very much.

Sour cream

Substitute plain nonfat Greek yogurt for sour cream. Thanks to the thick, creamy texture of Greek yogurt, you won't even miss the added fat. Works great for dips, salads and sauces.

Cheese

Switch from full-fat cheese to 50 percent light cheese or part-skim varieties to eliminate about half the saturated fat.

Salt

Although it is tempting to add salt to boost the flavor of a dish, instead look first to spices and herbs, such as basil, garlic powder, onion powder, oregano, parsley and rosemary.

1

Skinny-Size It Breakfast

Tempted to skip breakfast because you don't feel hungry in the morning? Think again! Studies continue to pile up that link eating breakfast to weighing less. Researchers have found that breakfast skippers engage in lower levels of physical activity and have a lower fruit and vegetable intake, and they have increased levels of fat and soft drink consumption—all factors that go against the Skinny Rules. Eating a higher amount of overall calories at breakfast is linked to lower weight gain in middle age. It is also interesting that in research studies, the groups that had the highest percentage of calories at breakfast had a higher total daily energy intake, yet they gained the least amount of weight. So forget just moving through your morning with a cup of coffee. Instead, work these Skinny–Size It breakfasts into your routine to fuel your body!

BREAKFAST BURRITOS

Yield: 4 servings

Before:

Grabbing a breakfast burrito at a restaurant can translate into consuming as much as or more than 30 grams of fat, 600 calories and 2,000 milligrams of sodium, which is nearly a day's worth of sodium.

Skinny Shopping:

Look for corn tortillas in the Mexican food aisle of your grocery store. Most corn tortillas only have around 10 milligrams of sodium. Remember to double-check the sodium content on the Nutrition Facts panel as it can vary greatly when making your selection. Many tortillas, especially flour tortillas, have 400 or more milligrams of sodium per tortilla! Salsa can be loaded with sodium too—opt for fresh salsas for the lowest sodium content, like Wholly Salsa, with only 25 milligrams of sodium per serving.

Skinny-Size It:
Fueling your body in the morning is essential, and whipping up this burrito takes only a matter of minutes. The filling is a mix of sautéed vegetables, whole eggs and egg whites, and it is wrapped up in a soft corn tortilla. It's then garnished with light toppings, like nonfat Greek yogurt, salsa and shredded light jalapeño cheese. You will be starting your day the Skinny way—with only a fraction of the calories, fat and sodium compared to the traditional breakfast burrito.

Skinny Cooking:

Sautéing is traditionally done with oil and/or butter, which adds calories and fat. Each tablespoon of oil adds 120 calories and 14 grams of fat to a recipe. The Skinny way is to sauté sans oil! Believe it or not, it actually works. Vegetables like onions and peppers have water in them which sweat as they are cooked and provide moisture to sauté. Another option is to prepare the pan with nonstick cooking spray, although cooking sprays are not truly calorie free or fat free; the first ingredient on the ingredient list is oil. Food labeling laws allow less than 5 calories or less than half grams of fat to round down to zero on the Nutrition Facts panel. So although cooking spray has fewer calories and less fat compared to pouring oil into a pan, when possible the skinniest way is to skip it all together!

Ingredients

½ cup diced sweet onion

½ cup diced red bell pepper

4 large eggs

4 large egg whites

8 small (6-inch) soft white corn tortillas

½ cup plain nonfat Greek yogurt

½ cup fresh tomato salsa of your choice

½ cup shredded light jalapeño cheddar cheese
(such as Cabot Jalapeño Light Cheddar Cheese)

Directions

1. Heat a medium skillet over medium heat. Sauté the onions and peppers until tender, about 3 to 5 minutes.

2. Add the whole eggs and the egg whites and scramble until they are cooked through. Remove the skillet from the heat.

3. Warm the tortillas in a microwave oven by placing them on a microwave-safe plate and covering them with a damp paper towel. Microwave them on high in 30-second intervals until they are warm and pliable.

4. Arrange the warmed tortillas on 4 individual plates. Spread yogurt, salsa and cheese on each, and then top with the egg-veggie mixture. Fold the tortillas in half, and serve at once.

Nutrition Facts (per serving)

300 calories, 9 grams fat, 3 grams saturated fat, 0 grams trans fat, 220 milligrams cholesterol, 400 milligrams sodium, 36 grams carbohydrates, 3 grams fiber, 4 grams sugar, 17 grams protein

EGG-LIKE BREAKFAST SCRAMBLE

Yield: 2 servings

Before:

Traditional egg scrambles are loaded with cholesterol. In just 3 eggs there are 558 milligrams of cholesterol, which is almost double the daily recommended heart-healthy limit of 300 milligrams. Plus, traditional egg scrambles pack around 300 calories or more.

Skinny-Size It:

The Egg-Like Breakfast Scramble contains only a third of the calories, thanks to exchanging the eggs for silken tofu. It also boasts 0 milligrams of cholesterol and only 110 calories. You even could add a slice of 100 percent whole-wheat toast and still consume fewer calories than are contained in a traditional egg scramble alone.

Skinny Shopping:

Like all tofu, silken tofu is made from soybeans. It has a softer, more delicate texture than regular tofu. At the store, you can find it in shelf-stable (aseptic) packaging or in the refrigerated section, near the rest of the tofu selections.

Ingredients

1 cup diced red bell pepper

½ cup diced sweet onion

8 ounces silken tofu, drained on paper towels

2 teaspoons garlic powder

2 teaspoons onion powder

Sea salt, to taste

Directions

1. Heat a medium skillet over medium heat. Sauté the peppers and onions until tender, about 3 to 5 minutes.

2. Add the tofu, garlic powder, onion powder and sea salt, and mix well. Cook for 8 to 10 minutes, or until the scramble is hot. Serve at once.

Nutrition Facts (per serving)

110 calories, 3.5 grams fat, 0 grams saturated fat, 0 grams trans fat, 0 milligrams cholesterol, 5 milligrams sodium, 15 grams carbohydrates, 2 grams fiber, 6 grams sugar, 7 grams protein

SKINNY SKILLET SCRAMBLE

Yield: 2 servings

Before:

Breakfast skillets are often loaded with calories and fat. When you order a breakfast skillet in a restaurant, it can have as much as 700 calories and 50 grams of fat.

Skinny-Size It:

Incorporating lots of vegetables and beans produces a more flavorful, lighter version of the breakfast skillet, without all the fat and calories. To make it even lighter, swap all the whole eggs for egg whites, since the yolk is where the majority of calories in an egg is stored. The white is a complete source of protein, yet it has only 15 calories. The Skinny Skillet Scramble has only 190 calories and 4 grams of fat per serving.

Ingredients

1 small red potato, diced

½ medium sweet onion, peeled and diced

½ medium red or green bell pepper, seeded, deribbed and diced

1 cup canned black beans, rinsed and drained

1 teaspoon garlic powder

4 large egg whites

2 large eggs

¼ cup shredded light cheddar cheese (such as Cabot Sharp Light Cheddar Cheese)

Directions

1. Heat a large skillet over medium heat. Sauté the potatoes, onions and peppers until all the vegetables have browned and are tender, about 7 minutes. Stir in the black beans and garlic powder and cook for 5 minutes more.

2. Add the egg whites and the whole eggs to the vegetable-bean mixture, and cook, stirring frequently, until the eggs have set, about 3 to 5 minutes.

3. Sprinkle the cheese over the scramble, cover the skillet and let the cheese melt, about 2 minutes. Serve at once.

Nutrition Facts (per serving)

190 calories, 4 grams fat, 1.5 grams saturated fat, 0 grams trans fat, 110 milligrams cholesterol, 150 milligrams sodium, 22 grams carbohydrates, 5 grams fiber, 4 grams sugar, 17 grams protein

APPLE QUINOA CRUNCH

Yield: 4 servings

While oatmeal is a great way to start the day, quinoa is a fabulous alternative to work into your breakfast lineup.

Before:

Many breakfast cereals have a lot of added sugar in the form of corn syrup or brown sugar.

Skinny-Size It:

This cereal features fresh fruit, diced apple, to sweeten your breakfast without adding sugar. In addition, the chopped almonds add crunch, healthy fat and flavor.

Skinny Shopping:

Quinoa is a seed that cooks up like a grain. It is a complete protein, because it has all the essential amino acids. Look for quinoa near the rice in your grocery store. It comes in red, white and purple/black varieties. Nutritionally, they are all the same, but the red variety tends to have a hint of sweetness.

Ingredients

1 cup cooked quinoa (⅓ cup dry)

2 medium McIntosh, Golden Delicious
(or other varieties good for cooking) apples,
peeled, cored and diced

1 ounce (about 22 nuts) unsalted almonds, chopped

1 teaspoon ground cinnamon

¼ cup low-fat milk or almond milk

Directions

1. Combine the quinoa, apples, almonds and cinnamon in a medium saucepan. Cook over medium heat, stirring frequently, for 3 to 5 minutes, or until the cereal is heated through.

2. Spoon the cereal into serving bowls, top with a tablespoon of milk, and serve at once.

Nutrition Facts (per serving)

120 calories, 4.5 grams fat, 0 grams saturated fat, 0 grams trans fat, 0 milligrams cholesterol, 10 milligrams sodium, 18 grams carbohydrates, 3 grams fiber, 7 grams sugar, 4 grams protein

OATMEAL OMEGA PARFAIT

Yield: 1 serving

Before:

Granola parfaits are often loaded with calories from sugar and sugary sweet granola. While they may contain some whole grains, when you really look at the nutrition details, is this really the best choice? Furthermore, traditional granola parfaits tend to leave you with a quick energy crash after the sugar rush.

Skinny-Size It:

Make your own parfait by layering oatmeal, fresh fruit, yogurt and Barlean's Strawberry Banana Omega Swirl Flax Oil.

This is a winning combination that will fill you up without the sugar rush and energy crash. Oatmeal Omega Parfait contains only 9 grams of sugar per serving, and the fiber and protein will help to keep you full and will help balance blood sugar levels, too.

Skinny Tip:

What is the difference between steel-cut oats and rolled oats? Steel-cut oats are whole-grain groats (grains of oat missing only the hull) that are cut into little pieces and when cooked have a heartier texture. Rolled oats (aka old-fashioned oats) are oat groats that have been steamed and rolled to reduce the cooking time. Nutritionally both are a great option but switch it up from time to time for the texture variety!

Ingredients

½ cup cooked steel-cut or old-fashioned oats (¼ cup dry oats)

½ cup sliced strawberries

½ cup plain nonfat Greek yogurt

1 tablespoon Barlean's Strawberry Banana Omega Swirl Flax Oil

Directions

1. In a clear 12-ounce or larger drinking glass, layer the oatmeal, sliced strawberries, yogurt and flax oil, alternating, up to the top of the glass. Serve at once.

Nutrition Facts (per serving)

230 calories, 7 grams fat, 1 gram saturated fat, 0 grams trans fat, 0 milligrams cholesterol, 55 milligrams sodium, 30 grams carbohydrates, 4 grams fiber, 9 grams sugar, 15 grams protein

TROPICAL MANGO OATMEAL

Yield: 2 servings

Before:

Many oatmeal recipes contain added sugar, which delivers sweetness but is not nutrient rich.

Skinny Shopping:

Coconut milk is typically found in the baking section and the ethnic food section of the grocery store. Regular coconut milk is high in calories and saturated fat, so the Skinny choice is light coconut milk. Not only does it have a lighter calorie price tag, but it is also full of flavor. In general, the goal is to limit the amount of saturated fat in your diet, though research is finding that not all saturated fats are created equal. For example, the saturated fat in coconut milk is lauric acid, which doesn't seem to adversely impact heart health.

Skinny-Size It:

To add sweetness to dishes, turn to fresh fruit. For example, this recipe derives its sweet taste from mango (a personal favorite), shredded coconut and light coconut milk, resulting in a tropical way to start your day. While the overall sugar content (14 grams per serving) is similar to that of plain oatmeal with a tablespoon of brown sugar, this recipe boasts 4 grams of fiber per serving, which is double the amount in plain oatmeal sweetened with brown sugar thanks to the mango. Plus, the mango provides immune-boosting vitamin A and vitamin C!

Ingredients

1 cup water

½ cup old-fashioned oats

1 cup diced mango

1 tablespoon shredded coconut

½ cup light coconut milk

Directions

1. Bring the water to a boil in a small saucepan over medium-high heat. Add the oats, reduce the heat to low and cook for 5 to 7 minutes, stirring frequently.
2. Spoon the oatmeal into 2 serving bowls. Top each bowl with the diced mango, shredded coconut and coconut milk, and serve at once.

Nutrition Facts (per serving)

160 calories, 4.5 grams fat, 2.5 grams saturated fat, 0 grams trans fat, 0 milligrams cholesterol, 15 milligrams sodium, 29 grams carbohydrates, 4 grams fiber, 14 grams sugar, 3 grams protein

BRAN FLAX MUFFINS

Yield: 12 servings (1 muffin each)

Before:

Store-bought muffins tend to be gigantic in size, and one muffin can have as much fat as you need for a whole day. In addition to their large size and fat content, they tend to be made with all-purpose white flour, which lacks fiber and other key nutrients.

Skinny-Size It:

Whole-wheat flour, flaxseed meal and wheat bran not only make a wonderful base for a muffin, but they also deliver fiber to help balance blood sugar levels and keep you feeling full! This muffin gains additional fiber from shredded carrots and apples and uses the Skinny swap of 4 egg whites, instead of 2 whole eggs.

Skinny Tip:

Flaxseed meal is made from flaxseeds, which are rich in omega-3 fatty acids and are high in fiber.

Ingredients

Nonstick cooking spray or 12 paper cupcake liners, for greasing or lining the muffin tin

1½ cups whole-wheat flour

1 cup brown sugar

¾ cup flaxseed meal

¾ cup wheat bran

2 teaspoons baking soda

1 teaspoon baking powder

2 teaspoons ground cinnamon

½ teaspoon sea salt

¾ cup low-fat milk

4 large egg whites, beaten

1 teaspoon vanilla extract

1½ cups shredded carrots

2 medium McIntosh, Golden Delicious (or other varieties good for baking) apples, peeled, cored and shredded

Directions

1. Preheat the oven to 350°F. Coat the wells of a 12-cup muffin tin with cooking spray or line the wells with paper cupcake liners.
2. In a large mixing bowl, combine the flour, brown sugar, flaxseed meal, wheat bran, baking soda, baking powder, cinnamon and sea salt, and mix thoroughly.
3. Make a well in the center of the dry mixture. Add the milk, egg whites and vanilla, and stir until well combined.
4. Fold in the shredded carrots and apples.
5. Spoon the batter into the wells of the prepared muffin tin, so that each well is about three-quarters full.
6. Bake for 15 to 20 minutes, or until a toothpick inserted in the middle of a muffin comes out clean.

Nutrition Facts (per serving)

170 calories, 3 grams fat, 0 grams saturated fat, 0 grams trans fat, 0 milligrams cholesterol, 430 milligrams sodium, 32 grams carbohydrates, 6 grams fiber, 16 grams sugar, 6 grams protein

WHOLE-WHEAT BLUEBERRY MUFFINS

Yield: 12 servings (1 muffin each)

Before:

Many fruit muffins gain their sweetness from added sugar and have only a small amount of actual fruit. Plus they are typically made with all-purpose white flour.

Skinny Swap:

Buttermilk actually contains no butter, as it is basically the sour milk that results from the curdling of the milk proteins and can have 5–8 grams of fat, or more, per cup. Buttermilk is used frequently in baking. Rather than buying buttermilk, make your own. Simply mix together 1 cup of low-fat milk and 1 tablespoon of white vinegar. Let it sit for about 3 to 5 minutes, and the proteins will begin to curdle. This homemade buttermilk recipe results in only 2.5 grams of fat per cup.

Skinny-Size It:

By switching from all-purpose white flour to whole-wheat flour and adding lots of fruit to these muffins, you end up with 3 grams of fiber in each muffin. Additionally, the recipe relies on the natural sweetness of fruit, thus eliminating the need for much added sugar.

Ingredients

Nonstick cooking spray or 12 paper cupcake liners, for greasing or lining the muffin tin

2 cups whole-wheat flour

$\frac{1}{2}$ cup sugar

2 teaspoons baking powder

1 teaspoon baking soda

$\frac{1}{2}$ teaspoon sea salt

$\frac{3}{4}$ cup low-fat milk plus 1 tablespoon white vinegar (buttermilk)

2 large egg whites, beaten

2 tablespoons melted unsalted margarine (such as Earth Balance Natural Buttery Spread) or butter

1 teaspoon vanilla extract

2 cups fresh or frozen blueberries

Directions

1. Preheat the oven to 400°F. Coat the wells of a 12-cup muffin tin with cooking spray or line the wells with paper cupcake liners.
2. In a large mixing bowl, combine the flour, sugar, baking powder, baking soda and sea salt, and mix thoroughly.
3. Make a well in the center of the dry mixture. Add the buttermilk, egg whites, margarine and vanilla, and stir until well combined.

4. Fold in the blueberries.
5. Spoon the batter into the wells of the prepared muffin tin, so that each well is about two-thirds full.
6. Bake for 20 to 23 minutes, or until a toothpick inserted in the middle of a muffin comes out clean.

Nutrition Facts (per serving)

130 calories, 2 grams fat, 0 grams saturated fat, 0 grams trans fat, 0 milligrams cholesterol, 410 milligrams sodium, 28 grams carbohydrates, 3 grams fiber, 12 grams sugar, 4 grams protein

CARROT CAKE MUFFINS

Yield: 24 servings (1 muffin each)

Before:

Carrot cake is traditionally a calorie-heavy, sugary dessert. An average-size slice of traditional carrot cake could have as many as or even more than 350 calories, 15 or more grams of fat and lots of added sugar.

Skinny-Size It:

Changing this traditional dessert to a muffin format and tweaking the ingredients transforms it into a great breakfast that will fuel your morning, with only 120 calories per muffin and 5 grams of fat (one-third the total fat of a typical version of the original dessert). This recipe contains nearly double the amount of shredded carrots found in typical carrot cake recipes and derives more natural sweetness from pineapple. In my first version of this recipe, I included a Skinny version of traditional heavy cream cheese frosting. However, my taste testers said the muffins were even better without it! The frosting recipe became a dip instead (see Whipped Pineapple Dip on page 153)!

Skinny Kitchen:

A quick and easy way to grate carrots is with a shredding blade in a food processor.

Ingredients

Nonstick cooking spray or 24 paper cupcake liners, for greasing or lining the muffin tin

1 cup sugar

½ cup canola oil

2 large eggs

2 teaspoons vanilla extract

2 cups whole-wheat flour

2 teaspoons baking soda

2 teaspoons baking powder

2 teaspoons ground cinnamon

3 cups grated carrots (6 to 8 medium carrots)

½ cup crushed pineapple, drained

Directions

1. Preheat the oven to 350°F. Coat the wells of a 24-cup muffin tin with cooking spray or line the wells with paper cupcake liners.
2. In a large mixing bowl, combine the sugar, oil, eggs and vanilla, and mix well.

3. In a separate bowl, mix the dry ingredients: flour, baking soda, baking powder and cinnamon, and stir until well combined. Add the dry mixture to the large bowl containing the sugar, oil and egg mixture, and stir until well combined.

4. Fold in the carrots and the pineapple.

5. Spoon the batter into the wells of the prepared muffin tin, so that each well is half full.

6. Bake for 15 to 17 minutes, or until a toothpick inserted in the middle of a muffin comes out clean.

Nutrition Facts (per serving)

120 calories, 5 grams fat, 0.5 grams saturated fat, 0 grams trans fat, 20 milligrams cholesterol, 160 milligrams sodium, 18 grams carbohydrates, 2 grams fiber, 10 grams sugar, 2 grams protein

APPLE MUFFINS

Yield: 12 servings (1 muffin each)

Before:

Say good-bye to oily muffins!

Skinny-Size It:

These muffins are moist without any added oil. The moisture in the muffins comes from shredded apples and applesauce. Switching from 2 whole eggs to 4 egg whites skims about 368 milligrams of cholesterol and 10 grams of fat from the recipe (since a large whole egg contains about 5 grams of fat), and using whole-wheat flour adds fiber along with vitamins and minerals.

Skinny Tip:

If you do not like the taste of whole-wheat flour, try white whole-wheat flour, which is milled from white wheat, a variety of wheat that is lighter in color and flavor than traditional red wheat yet delivers all the nutrition of whole wheat.

Ingredients

Nonstick cooking spray or 12 paper cupcake liners, for greasing or lining the muffin tin

1½ cups whole-wheat flour

2 teaspoons baking powder

½ teaspoon ground cinnamon

½ teaspoon sea salt

4 large egg whites, beaten

½ cup brown sugar

½ cup Applesauce (see recipe on page 149)

2 teaspoons vanilla extract

3 medium McIntosh, Golden Delicious (or other varieties good for baking) apples, peeled, cored and shredded

Directions

1. Preheat the oven to 350°F. Coat the wells of a 12-cup muffin tin with cooking spray or line the wells with paper cupcake liners.
2. In a large mixing bowl, whisk together the flour, baking powder, cinnamon and sea salt, and mix well.

3. Make a well in the center of the dry mixture. Add the egg whites, brown sugar, Applesauce and vanilla, and stir until well combined.
4. Fold in the apples.
5. Spoon the batter into the wells of the prepared muffin tin, so that it is evenly distributed.
6. Bake for 20 to 30 minutes, or until a toothpick inserted in the middle of a muffin comes out clean.

Nutrition Facts (per serving)

120 calories, 0 grams fat, 0 grams saturated fat, 0 grams trans fat, 0 milligrams cholesterol, 200 milligrams sodium, 26 grams carbohydrates, 3 grams fiber, 13 grams sugar, 3 grams protein

BLUEBERRY BUCKWHEAT PANCAKES

Yield: 6 servings (2 pancakes each)

Before:

Depending on how pancakes are made, you can wind up starting your day with a whole lot of empty calories, little to no fiber and lots of sugar from syrup.

Skinny-Size It:

These pancakes are half whole-wheat flour and half buckwheat flour, which mixes up the taste while still adhering to 100 percent whole grains. And for sweetness, this recipe calls for blueberries in the batter and my homemade Blueberry Maple Syrup (see recipe on page 155) as the topping.

Skinny Tip:

Although the word *buckwheat* would lead you to think that buckwheat is a grain, it is actually the fruit seeds of an herb, the buckwheat plant, though it is still considered to be part of the whole-grain family. The triangular-shaped seeds are ground into flour, which has a nutty flavor and is gluten free. Because of its strong flavor, buckwheat flour is typically mixed with other flours. Look for buckwheat flour in the grocery store baking aisle, near the all-purpose white flour, or check the health food section of the store for this flour.

Ingredients

¾ cup whole-wheat flour

¾ cup buckwheat flour

1 tablespoon sugar

1 teaspoon baking soda

½ teaspoon sea salt

1½ cups low-fat milk plus 1 tablespoon white vinegar (buttermilk)

2 large egg whites, beaten

1 cup fresh or frozen blueberries

Nonstick cooking spray, for greasing the skillet or griddle

½ cup Blueberry Maple Syrup (see recipe on page 155)

Directions

1. In a large mixing bowl, combine the whole-wheat flour, buckwheat flour, sugar, baking soda and sea salt, and mix well.
2. Make a well in the center of the dry mixture. Add the buttermilk and egg whites, and stir until well combined.
3. Fold in the blueberries.
4. Coat a large skillet or griddle with cooking spray and then heat it over medium heat.
5. Working in batches, ladle ¼ cup of the pancake batter onto the skillet or griddle. Cook until bubbles appear on the surface and the underside is golden brown, about 1 minute. Flip the pancake with a spatula and cook it on the other side, about 1 minute more. Repeat until all the batter has been used.
6. Serve the pancakes at once with the Blueberry Maple Syrup.

Nutrition Facts (per serving)

190 calories, 1.5 grams fat, 0 grams saturated fat, 0 grams trans fat, < 5 milligrams cholesterol, 450 milligrams sodium, 38 grams carbohydrates, 5 grams fiber, 18 grams sugar, 7 grams protein

VERY BANANA PANCAKES

Yield: 6 servings (2 pancakes each)

Before:

A serving of traditional pancakes can have as much as or even more than 400 calories, 80 milligrams of cholesterol and 38 grams of sugar, while offering only about 1 gram of fiber!

Skinny-Size It:

These Skinny-size pancakes allow you to have the same number of pancakes as in a typical serving but at a cost of only 300 calories, almost no cholesterol and little added sugars. Most of the sugar in these pancakes comes from the fresh bananas in the batter, and a serving contains 6 grams of belly-filling fiber, thanks to the combination of whole-wheat (or oat) flour and oatmeal!

Skinny Swap:

In any pancake, muffin or cookie recipe swap each whole egg for 2 egg whites. This single change will trim the recipe by 65 calories, 5 grams of fat and 186 milligrams of cholesterol. Additionally, instead of all-purpose white flour, use 100 percent whole-wheat or oat flour, found in the grocery store baking aisle.

Ingredients

¾ cup old-fashioned oats

1½ cups low-fat milk plus 1 tablespoon white vinegar (buttermilk)

¾ cup whole-wheat flour or oat flour

1½ teaspoons baking powder

¾ teaspoon baking soda

½ teaspoon ground cinnamon

½ teaspoon sea salt

2 large egg whites, lightly beaten

1 tablespoon packed brown sugar

2 medium bananas, plus 1 sliced for garnishing

Nonstick cooking spray, for greasing the skillet or griddle

$\frac{1}{2}$ cup Banana Maple Syrup (see recipe on page 154)

Directions

1. In a small bowl, soak the oats in $\frac{3}{4}$ cup of the buttermilk for 10 minutes.
2. In a large mixing bowl, combine the flour, baking powder, baking soda, cinnamon and sea salt, and mix thoroughly.
3. Make a well in the center of the dry mixture. Add the egg whites, brown sugar, the remaining $\frac{3}{4}$ cup of buttermilk and the oat-buttermilk mixture, and mix until just combined.
4. Mash 2 of the bananas and fold gently into the pancake batter.
5. Coat a large skillet or griddle with cooking spray and then heat it over medium heat.
6. Working in batches, ladle $\frac{1}{4}$ cup of the pancake batter onto the skillet or griddle. Cook until bubbles appear on the surface and the underside is golden brown, about 1 minute. Flip the pancake with a spatula and cook it on the other side, about 1 minute more. Repeat until all the batter has been used.
7. Garnish the pancakes with the banana slices and serve at once with the Banana Maple Syrup.

Nutrition Facts (per serving)

300 calories, 3 grams fat, 1 gram saturated fat, 0 grams trans fat, < 5 milligrams cholesterol, 520 milligrams sodium, 60 grams carbohydrates, 6 grams fiber, 26 grams sugar, 10 grams protein

2
.....

Sandwiches, Salads and Soups

andwiches, salads and soups can be perfect for lunch or dinner! When it comes to sandwiches, many traditional recipes pile on meat and cheese and then maybe add some vegetables. The Skinny-Size It way shifts the focus of the sandwich to the vegetables, including plenty of them, and lightens up on or even skips the meat and cheese. Another must is to use 100 percent whole-grain bread, rolls, pita and wraps, and to serve some sandwiches open-faced to cut down on the quantity of bread.

Although salads always have a health halo, they can have seven hundred calories or more and forty grams of fat or more! Typically, where salads go wrong is with the dressings and the toppings. Spinach, romaine lettuce and other salad greens are fat free and only have about ten calories per cup. But overdoing typical salad toppings, such heavy hitters as cheese, croutons, meat, fried chicken and sour cream, results in a calorie and fat pileup. Skinny-Size It salads maximize flavor with homemade dressings and plenty of flavorful vegetables while strategically adding in fat from healthier options, like nuts, seeds and avocados, reduced-fat cheeses (such as light cheddar cheese) or flavor-packed cheeses (such as blue cheese or feta), where a little goes a long way.

Soup may or may not be a healthy option. The soup recipes included in *Skinny-Size It* are slimmed-down versions of some "infamous" soups, like French onion soup and creamy tomato soup. It is possible to enjoy such flavorful soups without the high-calorie price tag.

Mix and match some of the sandwich, salad and soup recipes for a delicious Skinny meal that will fill your bowl and plate and satisfy your hunger.

SKINNIER SPIEDIE SANDWICH

Yield: 4 servings

Before:
The spiedie sandwich, which has its roots in upstate New York State and features grilled marinated chicken, beef, lamb or pork, is actually a healthy option, although spiedies are mostly served on Italian bread or rolls and often topped with heavy blue cheese salad dressing and oily sautéed peppers and onions.

Skinny-Size It:

Use whole-wheat flatbread and plenty of fresh veggies, and make your own spiedie marinade to keep the sodium in check, and the result will be a skinnier spiedie sandwich. And the biggest change . . . swap the chicken, beef, lamb or pork for cubed tofu. A unique property of tofu is that it absorbs the flavors of whatever it is marinated and cooked in. In this case the spiedie marinade gives the tofu tons of flavor. In fact, recently, we had friends over for dinner, and the tofu spiedies were gone before the chicken ones.

Skinny Tip:

Another delicious way to enjoy spiedie tofu is in a spiedie salad. To make the salad, start with dark leafy greens, top them with chopped vegetables and cooked spiedie tofu cubes, and then drizzle the salad with Ranch Dressing (see recipe on page 147).

Ingredients

8 ounces extra-firm tofu

1 cup Spiedie Marinade (see recipe on page 158)

Nonstick cooking spray, for greasing the skillet

4 whole-wheat flatbreads (such as Flatout Healthy Grain Flatbread)

1 cup shredded romaine lettuce

2 plum tomatoes, sliced

Directions

1. Remove the tofu from the package and drain the excess water by placing the tofu on a plate lined with paper towels and letting it sit for 15 to 20 minutes.

2. Cut the tofu into 1-inch cubes and place the cubes in a medium-size mixing bowl. Pour the Spiedie Marinade over the tofu and allow it to marinate for at least 30 minutes.

3. Lightly coat a medium-size skillet with cooking spray, and then heat the skillet over medium heat. Remove the tofu from the marinade with a slotted spoon and sauté it in the skillet, turning it gently with a spatula, until it has browned on all sides, about 20 to 30 minutes.

4. Arrange the flatbreads on 4 individual plates. Place the tofu cubes on one half of the flatbreads and then top with the shredded lettuce and tomato slices. Fold the flatbreads in half, and serve at once.

Nutrition Facts (per serving)

230 calories, 13 grams fat, 1.5 grams saturated fat, 0 grams trans fat, 0 milligrams cholesterol, 460 milligrams sodium, 21 grams carbohydrates, 11 grams fiber, 2 grams sugar, 17 grams protein

AVOCADO REUBENS

Yield: 4 servings

Before:

The customary reuben sandwich is piled high with corned beef and can have as much as or even more than 450 calories and 25 grams of fat and over half a day's worth of sodium per sandwich (1,300 milligrams) or more.

Skinny-Size It:

Substituting avocado slices and juicy tomato slices for the corned beef gives the sandwich a different feel, but it is still delicious and has 4 grams of belly-slimming monounsaturated fat, thanks to the avocado. Mixing up your own Guiltless Thousand Island Dressing (see recipe on page 160) helps to keep this sandwich in check, too, resulting in a reuben sandwich with only 310 calories and 12 grams of fat.

Ingredients

1 cup low-sodium sauerkraut

8 slices rye bread

1 medium ripe Hass avocado, halved, pit removed, peeled and sliced

1 large tomato, cut into 8 slices (or 16 thin slices)

¼ cup Guiltless Thousand Island Dressing (see recipe on page 160)

Directions

1. Heat the sauerkraut in a small saucepan over medium heat for 5 to 7 minutes, or until it is warmed through.
2. Toast the rye bread in a toaster oven.
3. Arrange the toasted slices of rye bread on 4 individual plates. Layer avocado and tomato slices on a bread

slice on each plate, and then top with the sauerkraut and the Guiltless Thousand Island Dressing. Place the second bread slice atop the sandwiches, and serve at once.

Nutrition Facts (per serving)

310 calories, 12 grams fat, 1.5 grams saturated fat, 0 grams trans fat, 0 milligrams cholesterol, 720 milligrams sodium, 43 grams carbohydrates, 8 grams fiber, 7 grams sugar, 9 grams protein

QUINOA-BEAN BURGERS

Yield: 4 servings

Before:

Burgers are typically a high-fat and low-fiber sandwich, and thus they do not make most Skinny food lists.

Skinny-Size It:

A bean- and whole-grain-based (quinoa) burger is an excellent way to have a burger without overdoing it when it comes to calories and fat, and each burger has 10 grams of belly filling fiber! Serving up this burger atop tomato slices instead of on a roll cuts down on calories and adds flavor. A slice of sweet onion and a drizzle of honey mustard lend even more flavor. Or if you'd prefer, you can serve these burgers on whole-wheat rolls.

Skinny Tip:

When you are making quinoa, make a big batch and then store it in the refrigerator for up to 7 days. This way you can quickly serve it for breakfast or as a side dish to go with meals.

Ingredients

One 15 1/2-ounce can pinto beans, rinsed and drained

1 cup cooked quinoa (about 1/3 cup dry)

1/2 cup minced red bell pepper

1/4 cup minced sweet onion

1/4 cup whole-wheat panko bread crumbs

2 large egg whites

1 clove garlic, peeled and minced

Nonstick cooking spray, for greasing the skillet

1 large tomato, cut into 8 slices

1/2 large sweet onion, peeled and sliced thin

2 teaspoons honey mustard

Directions

1. Puree the pinto beans in a food processor until smooth. If necessary, add 1 teaspoon water to the beans to make a smooth puree.

2. In a large mixing bowl, combine the bean puree, quinoa, peppers, minced onion, bread crumbs,

egg whites and garlic. Mix well. Using your hands works best. Form the bean-quinoa mixture into 4 burgers.

3. Lightly coat a large skillet with cooking spray and cook the burgers over medium heat until warmed through, about 3 to 4 minutes per side.

4. Place the burgers atop the tomato slices, garnish with sweet onions, drizzle the honey mustard on top, and serve at once.

Nutrition Facts (per serving)

220 calories, 1.5 grams fat, 0 grams saturated fat, 0 grams trans fat, 0 milligrams cholesterol, 55 milligrams sodium, 40 grams carbohydrates, 10 grams fiber, 3 grams sugar, 13 grams protein

FLANK STEAK SANDWICH

Yield: 4 servings

Before:

Steak sandwiches, which are often loaded with cheese, can have 700 or more calories and upwards of 40 grams of fat per sandwich. Often they are served with a pile of fries too!

Skinny-Size It:

Make an open-faced steak sandwich with trimmed flank steak and top it with tons of sautéed peppers and onions and only some cheese for a much healthier version, and pair it with a Deliciously Skinny Side (see recipes on pages 97–126).

Skinny Tip:

Swiss cheese is naturally lower in sodium, with only about 50 milligrams per ounce compared to other cheeses that have as much as 175 milligrams per ounce. Plus, it is a perfect option for Skinny dishes because it is full of flavor, which means you can maximize the flavor of a dish while skimping on the amount of cheese used.

Ingredients

1 pound flank steak, fat trimmed

1 teaspoon garlic powder

$\frac{1}{2}$ teaspoon freshly cracked black pepper

1 medium red bell pepper, seeded, deribbed and sliced thin

1 medium green bell pepper, seeded, deribbed and sliced thin

1 large sweet onion, peeled and sliced thin

$\frac{1}{4}$ cup shredded Swiss cheese

2 whole-wheat (6-inch) sub rolls, cut in half

Directions

1. Preheat the grill.
2. Arrange the flank steak on a plate. In a small bowl, combine the garlic powder and black pepper. Rub the spice mix over the flank steak.

3. Grill the steak for 5 to 6 minutes per side, or until it reaches the desired doneness.

4. Remove the steak from the grill, place it on a clean plate, cover with aluminum foil, and allow it to sit for 10 minutes. Then transfer the steak to a cutting board and cut it diagonally into thin slices.

5. Heat a large skillet over medium heat. Sauté the red and green peppers and the onions until tender, 7 to 10 minutes. Sprinkle the cheese over the peppers and onions, cover the skillet, and cook until the cheese has melted, about 3 minutes.

6. Place the roll halves on a baking sheet and toast them under a low broiler until lightly browned, about 1 minute.

7. Arrange the toasted roll halves on 4 individual plates. Top each with the grilled steak slices and the pepper-onion mixture, and serve at once.

Nutrition Facts (per serving)

240 calories, 8 grams fat, 3.5 grams saturated fat, 0 grams trans fat, 35 milligrams cholesterol, 200 milligrams sodium, 19 grams carbohydrates, 3 grams fiber, 5 grams sugar, 24 grams protein

BBQ TEMPEH SANDWICH

Yield: 4 servings

Before:

Barbecue sandwiches tend to be made with pulled pork, which can be high in calories (600 calories or more per sandwich) and fat. Plus, many versions are loaded with sodium (1,200 milligrams or more).

Skinny-Size It:

Swap the pork for tempeh, which is made from cultured soybeans. Some varieties of tempeh, such as Lightlife Organic Three Grain Tempeh, are made with cultured soybeans with a blend of whole grains, like brown rice, barley and millet. By itself, tempeh has a light flavor, and so it works well when paired with flavorful sauces, such as Maple BBQ Sauce (see recipe on page 156).

Skinny Tip:

Try eating meatless on Monday! Tempeh is an excellent meat substitute. By eating meatless even once a week, you can reduce your risk for heart disease, diabetes, obesity and certain types of cancer. Check out www.meatlessmonday.com for more information and for tips on getting started!

Ingredients

2 cups sliced sweet onion

One 8-ounce package tempeh (such as Lightlife Organic Three Grain Tempeh), cut into ½-inch-thick slices

¼ cup Maple BBQ Sauce (see recipe on page 156)

4 slices 100 percent whole-wheat bread

Directions

1. Heat a large skillet over medium heat. Sauté the onions until tender, about 5 to 7 minutes. Remove the skillet from the heat and set aside.

2. While the onions are cooking, place the tempeh in a single layer in a small skillet and spread the Maple BBQ Sauce over it. Cook the tempeh over medium heat until heated through, about 5 to 7 minutes.

3. Toast the bread in a toaster oven.

4. Arrange the toast on 4 individual plates. Place the tempeh and the onions on top, and serve at once.

Nutrition Facts (per serving)

240 calories, 7 grams fat, 1.5 grams saturated fat, 0 grams trans fat, 0 milligrams cholesterol, 290 milligrams sodium, 33 grams carbohydrates, 3 grams fiber, 10 grams sugar, 14 grams protein

STACKED ALT SANDWICH

Yield: 2 servings

Before:

A typical BLT sandwich is high in fat—the majority of it is saturated fat—and just a few grams of fiber.

Skinny-Size It:

Preparing this nutrient-packed sandwich is so simple. It is filled with whole-grain ingredients, which means that a single sandwich has over half the daily recommended amount of fiber (the daily fiber goal is at least 25 grams) and 45 percent of the daily value for vitamin A and 50 percent of the daily value for vitamin C.

Skinny Shopping:

Don't be fooled in the bread aisle of the grocery store. While there are many whole-wheat-looking products, when you look closer at the ingredients list, you won't find that whole wheat is the first ingredient. Instead, you may find ingredients such as caramel color, which makes the bread look more like wheat bread. The best bet is to opt for 100 percent whole-wheat or whole white wheat breads and/or breads with other whole grains, like brown rice, listed as the first ingredient.

Ingredients

4 slices 100 percent whole-wheat bread

1 medium ripe Hass avocado, halved, pit removed, peeled and sliced thin

1 large tomato, cut into 8 thin slices

8 romaine lettuce leaves

¼ cup Ranch Dressing (see recipe on page 147)

Directions

1. Toast the whole-wheat bread and arrange the toasted slices on 2 individual plates.

2. Stack the avocado slices, tomato slices and lettuce leaves on one of the toasted slices. Spoon the Ranch Dressing over the top. Place the second toasted slice atop the sandwiches, and serve at once.

Nutrition Facts (per serving)

410 calories, 19 grams fat, 2 grams saturated fat, 0 grams trans fat, 0 milligrams cholesterol, 430 milligrams sodium, 55 grams carbohydrates, 14 grams fiber, 9 grams sugar, 12 grams protein

HUMMUS-CUCUMBER FLATBREAD

Yield: 1 serving

Before:

A flatbread sandwich from a drive-through can have more than 300 calories and 10 grams of fat or more.

Skinny-Size It:

In minutes you can make your own flatbread sandwich with hummus and cucumbers. This one has just 140 calories and boasts 10 grams of filling fiber. If you are on the go, try wrapping up the flatbread in wax paper and then placing it in a container or wrapping it with foil. This sandwich is so versatile, it can be sliced into small wedges and served as an appetizer. And it even tastes great for breakfast!

Ingredients

2 tablespoons Skinny-Size It Hummus (see recipe on page 148) or store-bought roasted red pepper hummus

1 whole-wheat flatbread (such as Flatout Soft 100% Whole Wheat Flatbread)

½ cup sliced cucumbers

1 teaspoon honey mustard

Directions

1. Spread the hummus evenly over the flatbread. Top with the cucumber slices and a drizzle of honey mustard.

Nutrition Facts (per serving)

140 calories, 4 grams fat, 0 grams saturated fat, 0 grams trans fat, 0 milligrams cholesterol, 470 milligrams sodium, 24 grams carbohydrates, 10 grams fiber, 2 grams sugar, 10 grams protein

ROASTED BEET AND RADICCHIO SALAD

Yield: 4 servings

Before:

The idea for this recipe came from a roasted beet salad that I had at a restaurant. The salad had the misfortune of swimming in dressing and being loaded down with cheese and caramelized pecans. It had to be loaded with calories, fat, sodium and sugar given all the dressing, cheese and sugary pecans.

Skinny-Size It:

Revamping the salad involved switching to toasted walnuts—toasting enhances the walnut's flavor and provides crunch without the added sugar—and then topping the salad with plenty of beets and some cheese to keep the calories in check. The salad is finished with my homemade Creamy Balsamic Dressing (see recipe on page 163), which is full of flavor and gets its silkiness from pureed cashews. Each serving of the revamped salad has only 160 calories, 7 grams of fat and 7 grams of fiber.

Skinny Tip:

Using heavy flavored cheeses like feta or blue cheese that deliver a strong flavor allows you to get away with adding smaller amounts of cheese, thus saving added calories and fat.

Ingredients

Aluminum foil, for roasting the beets

4 medium red, golden or multicolored beets, peeled and cut into ½-inch cubes

2 tablespoons walnuts

1 small head radicchio, shredded thin (sauté shredded radicchio until tender, about 5 to 7 minutes, if preferred)

¼ cup crumbled feta cheese or blue cheese

¼ cup Creamy Balsamic Dressing (see recipe on page 163)

Directions

1. Preheat the oven to 425°F. Line a baking sheet with aluminum foil.

2. Arrange the cubed beets on the foil-lined baking sheet and then place a sheet of aluminum foil over them, folding the edges to seal. Roast the beets in the oven until they are tender, about 45 to 50 minutes.

3. Heat a small skillet over medium heat, and add the walnuts. Cook the walnuts for 2 to 3 minutes, stirring frequently, or until they are lightly toasted.

4. Place the radicchio in 4 salad bowls. Arrange the roasted beets, the cheese and the toasted walnuts atop the radicchio. Drizzle the Creamy Balsamic Dressing over the salad, and serve at once.

Nutrition Facts (per serving)

160 calories, 7 grams fat, 2 grams saturated fat, 0 grams trans fat, 0 milligrams cholesterol, 200 milligrams sodium, 21 grams carbohydrates, 7 grams fiber, 13 grams sugar, 7 grams protein

SWEET POTATO AND BLUE SPINACH SALAD

Yield: 4 side salads or 2 entrée salads

Before:

An entrée-size spinach salad at a restaurant could have as much as 1,000 calories, 60-plus grams of fat and 1,000 or more milligrams of sodium.

Skinny Tip:

Combining colorful fruits and vegetables in this salad is a great way to keep the calories low while gaining sweetness and fiber. To boost the protein content of this salad, add sliced grilled chicken or tofu.

Skinny-Size It:

Putting together spinach salad at home allows you to control the amounts of the ingredients, and making your own dressing is a Skinny must. The result is significant calorie, fat and sodium savings. The entrée version of this salad has only 240 calories, 9 grams of fat and 250 milligrams of sodium per serving.

Ingredients

3 small sweet potatoes, peeled and cut into
   $1/4$-inch cubes

1 teaspoon extra-virgin olive oil

3 $1/2$ cups baby spinach, dried with a salad spinner

1 cup fresh blueberries

2 ounces blue cheese, crumbled

$1/2$ cup Creamy Balsamic Dressing (see recipe on page 163)

Directions

1. Preheat the oven to 425°F. Arrange the sweet potato cubes on a baking sheet or in a baking dish. Sprinkle the olive oil over the sweet potatoes and toss to coat, or spray them evenly with an oil mister.

2. Bake the sweet potatoes until they are lightly browned and tender, about 25 to 30 minutes, stirring occasionally throughout the baking process.

3. Arrange the spinach on a serving platter and top with the sweet potatoes, blueberries and blue cheese.

4. Immediately before serving the salad, warm the Creamy Balsamic Dressing in a microwave oven, and thin it, if necessary, by adding 1 to 2 teaspoons of water.

5. Drizzle the dressing over the salad, and serve at once.

Nutrition Facts (per side serving)

120 calories, 4.5 grams fat, 2 grams saturated fat, 0 grams trans fat, 5 milligrams cholesterol, 125 milligrams sodium, 17 grams carbohydrates, 3 grams fiber, 7 grams sugar, 4 grams protein

CREAMY CUCUMBER-TOMATO SALAD

Yield: 6 servings

Before:

The original version of this salad was my Grandma's, which had a dressing that was heavy on the sugar and was made with regular, full-fat mayonnaise.

Skinny Cooking:

When preparing cucumbers, it is best to leave the skin of the cucumber on because the skin has fiber and vitamins. Yet, most cucumbers in the grocery store have a wax coating. To eat cucumbers whole without worrying about a wax coating, opt for European cucumbers, which are typically shrink wrapped and never waxed. Or, when cucumbers are in season, buy them from a farmers' market and they will likely not be waxed. Then scrub the cucumber well before slicing!

Skinny-Size It:

Cutting back on the sugar and swapping full-fat mayonnaise for reduced-fat mayonnaise lightens up the dressing. The end result is a lighter version of the salad that is perfect for summer, with only 100 calories and 3 grams of fat per serving.

Ingredients

2 medium cucumbers, sliced

2 medium tomatoes, cut into 8 wedges each

1 large sweet onion, peeled and sliced thin

½ cup reduced-fat mayonnaise

¼ cup white vinegar

¼ cup sugar or agave nectar

½ teaspoon freshly cracked black pepper

Directions

1. Place the cucumbers, tomatoes and onions in a large serving bowl.
2. In a small mixing bowl, combine the mayonnaise, vinegar, sugar and black pepper, and whisk, mixing well.
3. Pour the dressing over the salad and toss to coat. Serve at once.

Nutrition Facts (per serving)

100 calories, 3 grams fat, 0 grams saturated fat, 0 grams trans fat, 0 milligrams cholesterol, 170 milligrams sodium, 18 grams carbohydrates, 1 gram fiber, 12 grams sugar, 1 gram protein

GRILLED PEAR AND SPINACH SALAD

Yield: 4 servings

Before:

Many salads, especially those at restaurants, start with a base of chopped iceburg lettuce, which is low in calories but low in nutrient value too.

Skinny Tip:

There are four vitamins that are fat soluble, which means your body will not be able to absorb them without some fat present in your food. They are vitamin A, vitamin D, vitamin E and vitamin K. This is the primary reason to avoid making your salads completely fat free.

Skinny-Size It:

Keeping in mind that food is fuel, you may as well maximize the types of foods and make them nutrient rich. A bed of dark greens, such as spinach, is a great nutrient-rich base for any salad. Toppings that maximize the salad's flavor and increase its nutritional benefits are a must. For example, the toppings for this salad are mostly fruits and nuts. The walnuts add heart-helping omega-3 fatty acids and crunch, and the dried cranberries and the grilled pears impart sweetness and excellent flavor. When it comes to cheese, skimp on the portion to keep the calories and saturated fat content of the salad in check—each serving of this salad only has 2.5 grams of saturated fat total!

Ingredients

1 ripe pear, halved, cored and then cut into $\frac{1}{2}$-inch-thick slices

$\frac{1}{2}$ cup walnuts

4 cups baby spinach, dried with a salad spinner

$\frac{1}{2}$ cup dried cranberries

$\frac{1}{4}$ cup crumbled blue cheese

$\frac{1}{4}$ cup White Balsamic Vinaigrette (see recipe on page 151)

Directions

1. Preheat the grill. Place the pear slices directly onto the hot grill, and grill them on each side for 2 to 4 minutes, or until they have grill marks.
2. Heat a small skillet over medium heat, and add the walnuts. Cook the walnuts for 2 to 3 minutes, stirring frequently, or until they are lightly toasted.
3. Arrange the spinach in a large serving bowl, and top with the grilled pear slices, the toasted walnuts, the cranberries and the blue cheese. Drizzle the White Balsamic Vinaigrette over the salad, and serve at once.

Nutrition Facts (per serving)

240 calories, 15 grams fat, 2.5 grams saturated fat, 0 grams trans fat, 5 milligrams cholesterol, 190 milligrams sodium, 23 grams carbohydrates, 3 grams fiber, 15 grams sugar, 7 grams protein

GRILLED PANZANELLA SALAD

Yield: 8 servings

Before:

The idea for this recipe is inspired for a favorite dish of mine at a local restaurant. The original version has grilled chicken and feta cheese in it, as well.

Skinny-Size It:

Making the Honey Vinaigrette (see recipe on page 159) from scratch keeps the sodium level of this salad under control. This dressing is an excellent marinade for the vegetables. Another key to this recipe is grilling the vegetables after roasting them, as grilling increases their sweetness, especially that of the peppers and onions. Each serving of this salad has only 130 calories and 5 grams of fat.

Skinny Shopping:

Capers are the tiny dark green immature flower buds of the caper bush. They resemble green peas somewhat but taste something like olives since they are pickled in a vinegar brine. You will find them typically near the olives on the grocery store shelf. Their tangy flavor works perfectly for salads, and they are excellent with smoked salmon. You can also find larger capers, sometimes called caper berries, which are actually the matured fruit of the caper bush and are about the size of an olive.

Ingredients

2 medium yellow bell peppers, seeded, deribbed and
cut into 1-inch pieces

1 medium red bell pepper, seeded, deribbed and cut
into 1-inch pieces

1 medium green bell pepper, seeded, deribbed and
cut into 1-inch pieces

1 medium cucumber, seeded and cut into 1-inch pieces

1 pint cherry tomatoes

1 small sweet onion, peeled and cut into 1-inch pieces

1 cup Honey Vinaigrette (see recipe on page 159), divided

1 teaspoon extra-virgin olive oil

2 whole-wheat rolls or 4 slices 100 percent whole-wheat
bread, cut into 1-inch pieces

1 teaspoon garlic powder

2 tablespoons capers, rinsed and drained

Directions

1. Preheat the oven to 350°F.
2. In a large mixing bowl, combine the yellow, red and
   green peppers, cucumbers, tomatoes and onions.
   Pour ½ cup of the Honey Vinaigrette over the
   vegetables and toss gently to coat.
3. Divide the vegetables evenly between 2 baking
   sheets, and roast them in the oven for 15 to
   20 minutes, or until they are warmed through
   yet still slightly crispy. Remove the vegetables from
   the oven and set aside.
4. Heat the grill to low heat. Place the roasted vegetables
   in a grill basket and lightly grill them for 5 minutes.
5. Heat the olive oil in a large skillet over medium heat.
   Add the bread and cook for 5 minutes, turning the

bread frequently so that it browns evenly.
Then sprinkle the garlic powder over the croutons
and toss to coat.

6. Arrange the grilled vegetables on a large serving
platter, and top with the croutons and capers.
Drizzle the salad with the remaining ½ cup of
Honey Vinaigrette, and serve warm or chilled.

Nutrition Facts (per serving)

130 calories, 5 grams fat, 0.5 grams saturated fat, 0 grams trans
fat, 0 milligrams cholesterol, 160 milligrams sodium, 18 grams
carbohydrates, 2 grams fiber, 7 grams sugar, 3 grams protein

MIXED-UP COBB SALAD

Yield: 4 servings

Before:

Cobb salads are loaded with heavy hitter toppings like
cheese, egg, avocado and bacon. Restaurant versions can
have 500 calories or more, upwards of 35 grams of fat and
15 grams of saturated fat—which is an entire day's worth of
saturated fat.

Skinny-Size It:

Making your own Mixed-Up Cobb Salad is pretty simple.
This recipe preserves the traditional Cobb flavors and even
includes a little bacon! One fundamental distinction is that
this Cobb salad is loaded with veggies including corn, red
and orange bell peppers, onions and avocado. It is essential to make your own salad dressing for this salad. Both
Creamy Balsamic Dressing (see recipe on page 163) and

Ranch Dressing (see recipe on page 147) work perfectly with this recipe. The final tally for this filling Cobb salad is 250 calories and 14 grams of fat per serving, plus 8 grams of fiber and only 170 milligrams of sodium.

Skinny Tip:

When dining in restaurants it is wise to order salad dressings on the side because you can't be certain how much dressing the chef will add to your salad. When making salads at home, you can toss salad toppings that are not too delicate with dressing. This technique spreads the dressing's flavor throughout the salad while minimizing the amount of added dressing. Just keep in mind that too much of even the healthiest of dressings can unravel any swaps you have made in a recipe.

Ingredients

1 cup fresh or frozen corn, cooked and drained

1 medium ripe Hass avocado, halved, pit removed, peeled and chopped

1 small red bell pepper, seeded, deribbed and diced

1 small orange bell pepper, seeded, deribbed and diced

½ small red onion, peeled and diced

2 slices center-cut bacon, cooked until crisp and crumbled

¼ cup crumbled blue cheese

¼ cup Creamy Balsamic Dressing (see recipe on page 163) or Ranch Dressing (see recipe on page 147)

4 cups chopped romaine lettuce or baby spinach

Directions

1. In a large mixing bowl, combine the corn, avocado, red and orange bell peppers, onions, bacon and blue cheese. Pour the Creamy Balsamic Dressing or Ranch Dressing over the vegetables and toss gently to coat.

2. Arrange the romaine lettuce or spinach in 4 serving bowls and spoon the vegetables coated with dressing on top. Serve at once.

Nutrition Facts (per serving)

250 calories, 14 grams fat, 4 grams saturated fat, 0 grams trans fat, 10 milligrams cholesterol, 170 milligrams sodium, 25 grams carbohydrates, 8 grams fiber, 7 grams sugar, 8 grams protein

VEGGIE CHILI

Yield: 12 servings

Before:

Chili is a hearty stew that can have 8 grams of fat or more per serving from beef, oil and other sources. Plus it is often topped with full-fat shredded cheese and sour cream.

Skinny-Size It:

Made completely from vegetables and beans, Veggie Chili has a slim 1 gram of fat per serving and 8 grams of fiber per serving. The chili powder listed in the ingredient list is to taste, as the amount added to the dish definitely depends on the audience you are cooking for and how spicy they can tolerate their foods. Since our little guys like some spice but not too much, I leave it out of the chili and then add it to individual serving dishes before serving.

Skinny Tip:

An even skinnier way to make this recipe is to use dried beans that you've soaked overnight, which will even further cut down on the amount of sodium in the dish! Canned beans are certainly a time saver, and rinsing and draining the beans eliminates about 41 percent of the sodium content.

Ingredients

Two 15 ½ ounce cans kidney beans, rinsed and drained

One 15 ½ ounce can cannellini or pinto beans, rinsed and drained

One 14 ½ ounce can diced tomatoes

2 cups low-sodium vegetable broth

2 cups fresh or frozen corn

1 ½ cups diced sweet onion

1 cup fresh mild salsa of your choice

½ large red bell pepper, seeded, deribbed and chopped (about 1 cup)

Chili powder, to taste

Sea salt, to taste

Directions

1. Combine all the ingredients except the chili powder and the sea salt in a slow cooker. Cook on low for 6 to 8 hours. If you do not have a slow cooker, combine all the ingredients in a large soup pot, bring to a boil over medium-high heat, and then lower the heat and simmer for 1 hour.

2. Season the chili with chili powder and sea salt to taste, and serve at once.

Nutrition Facts (per serving)

180 calories, 1 gram fat, 0 grams saturated fat, 0 grams trans fat, 0 milligrams cholesterol, 250 milligrams sodium, 35 grams carbohydrates, 8 grams fiber, 4 grams sugar, 10 grams protein

FRENCH ONION SOUP

Yield: 6 servings

Before:

A bowl of classic French onion soup commonly harbors over 200 calories per serving and 15 grams of fat, thanks to the thick layer of cheese baked on top of the soup.

Skinny-Size It:

Instead of having lots of cheese baked on top, this version of French Onion Soup features a slice of whole-wheat baguette or roll that has been sprinkled with a modest amount of shredded Swiss cheese, placed under the broiler and then floated in the soup. Using a low-sodium broth allows you to lower the amount of added sodium in the soup. The Skinny-Size It version of French Onion Soup has only 120 calories and 2 grams of fat per serving.

Skinny Tip:

A cousin of mine loves to tell the story of watching me prepare soup in which I used low-sodium broth and then (his exaggerated description) poured tons of salt in at the end. Using low-sodium broth is always the best bet, because then you can minimize the amount of sodium in the soup. And no, I would never pour tons of salt in a dish. But starting with low-sodium broth allows you to better control the sodium content, even if you add some salt at the end. Remember to measure the amount of salt you add to a dish to keep the sodium level in check. And remember that just 1 teaspoon of salt has about 2,300 milligrams of sodium.

Ingredients

2 large sweet onions, peeled and diced

2 cloves garlic, peeled and minced

2 tablespoons all-purpose white flour

1 teaspoon sugar

½ teaspoon dried parsley

½ teaspoon dried thyme

½ teaspoon freshly ground black pepper

4 cups low-sodium beef or vegetable broth

1 cup dry white wine

Sea salt, to taste

6 ½ inch-thick slices whole-wheat baguette or
    whole-wheat roll

¼ cup grated Swiss cheese

Directions

1. Heat a large soup pot over medium heat. Sauté the
    onions and the garlic until they have lightly browned,
    about 10 minutes.

2. Add the flour and the sugar to the onions, stir well,
    and cook over medium heat, until golden brown.
    Then add the parsley, thyme and black pepper.

3. Add the broth and the wine, bring to a boil, and
    then lower the heat and simmer the soup for
    45 minutes. Add sea salt to taste.

4. Preheat the broiler to low. Place the baguette slices
    (or whole-wheat rolls) on a baking sheet. Toast the
    baguette slices under the broiler for 1 minute, or
    until they have browned. (Note: If you are not
    serving all the soup at once, toast only those
    baguette slices you will be using and reserve the
    rest for toasting later.)

5. Top the baguette slices with Swiss cheese, return
    them to the oven, and broil until the cheese is
    melted, about 1 to 2 minutes.

6. Assemble the soup by placing a broiled baguette
    slice in each of 6 individual serving bowls. Ladle
    the soup over the baguette, and serve at once.

Nutrition Facts (per serving)

120 calories, 2 grams fat, 1 gram saturated fat, 0 grams trans fat, 0 milligrams cholesterol, 170 milligrams sodium, 18 grams carbohydrates, 2 grams fiber, 4 grams sugar, 5 grams protein

MINESTRONE SOUP

Yield: 12 servings (1 cup each)

Before:

Traditional minestrone soup has meat or a combination of meats (such as ground beef and bacon or pancetta), added fat from the olive oil used to sauté the vegetables, non-whole-wheat pasta and added salt. The per serving calorie total winds up being over 200 calories, and the soup customarily contains 8 grams of fat or more.

Skinny-Size It:

Skipping the oil and sweating the vegetables in a skillet, skipping the meat, and increasing the quantity of vegetables—including kicking up the dark leafy greens—results in a hearty soup with only 150 calories and 1.5 grams of fat per serving.

Ingredients

1 large sweet onion, peeled and diced

3 large carrots, peeled and chopped

4 cloves garlic, peeled and minced

One 28-ounce can diced tomatoes with Italian herbs

2 cups low-sodium vegetable broth

One 15 ½ ounce can kidney beans, drained and rinsed

One 15½ ounce can black beans, drained
and rinsed

4 cups chopped baby spinach

¼ cup dry whole-wheat rotini pasta

½ teaspoon white pepper

½ cup grated Parmesan cheese

Directions

1. Sweat the onions in a large soup pot over medium heat, stirring frequently, until they are translucent, about 5 to 10 minutes.

2. Add the carrots and garlic, and sweat until just fragrant, about 3 minutes.

3. Add the tomatoes, broth, kidney beans and black beans, and bring to a boil.

4. Add the spinach, whole-wheat pasta and white pepper. Bring to a boil, reduce the heat, cover and simmer the soup for 10 to 12 minutes, or until the pasta and the carrots are cooked.

5. Ladle the soup into individual serving bowls, sprinkle the grated Parmesan cheese on top, and serve at once.

Nutrition Facts (per serving)

150 calories, 1.5 grams fat, 0.5 grams saturated fat, 0 grams trans fat, < 5 milligrams cholesterol, 330 milligrams sodium, 27 grams carbohydrates, 6 grams fiber, 4 grams sugar, 9 grams protein

CREAMY GARLIC TOMATO SOUP

Yield: 4 servings

Before:

Creamy soups tend to fall in the loaded category when it comes to calories and fat.

Skinny-Size It:

Prepare this Skinny-Size It creamy soup by starting with a super simple and creamy white sauce as the base! The white sauce is made with low-fat milk or unsweetened almond milk and derives all its flavor from the garlic and the tomatoes. Each serving of this soup has only 120 calories, 3 grams of fat and 80 milligrams of sodium.

Skinny Swap:

Use unsweetened almond milk in place of low-fat milk and save 60 calories per cup. Plus, almond milk has 0 grams of saturated fat and provides 1.5 grams of monounsaturated fat per cup. You can find unsweetened almond milk near the dairy section or in the health food section of your grocery store. There are several varieties of almond milk on the market, so be certain to choose the unsweetened variety, which works best for cooking.

Ingredients

1 tablespoon unsalted butter

1 tablespoon all-purpose white flour

2 cloves garlic, peeled and minced

1 1/2 teaspoons garlic powder

1 cup low-fat milk or unsweetened almond milk

3 cups canned tomatoes (with juice)

Directions

1. Melt the butter in a medium-size soup pot over medium heat. Once the butter has melted, whisk in the flour. Then whisk in the garlic and garlic powder.

2. Add the milk and whisk frequently until the mixture is bubbly, about 5 minutes. Cook for 1 minute more, or until the sauce thickens.

3. Add the tomatoes to the sauce and cook for 7 to 10 minutes, or until the soup is hot.

4. Using an immersion blender, puree the soup until it is smooth, or puree in a blender or food processor until smooth. (If using a blender, remove the center piece from the top of the blender and cover the hole with a cloth, since the pressure can cause the top to fly off when blending, making a huge mess. I have made that mistake before!) Serve the soup at once.

Nutrition Facts (per serving)

120 calories, 3 grams fat, 0.5 grams saturated fat, 0 grams trans fat, < 5 milligrams cholesterol, 80 milligrams sodium, 18 grams carbohydrates, 4 grams fiber, 9 grams sugar, 5 grams protein

3
....

Healthy
Entrées

Almost half the entrée recipes in this chapter are vegetarian and include plenty of vegetables! And the nonvegetarian entrées, such as Meat Loaf Muffins, Traditional General Tso's Chicken and Cheesy Chicken, contain vegetables and/or fruits in larger quantities than is found in traditional versions of these dishes. Although the protein portion sizes of these entrées may seem small at first, they are actually just right given that a four-ounce piece of meat supplies about twenty-eight grams of protein. Incorporating lots of fruits and vegetables into the entrées makes the overall portions larger, so you don't feel like you have a tiny piece of chicken or meat sitting on your plate.

RETHINKING HOW YOU FILL YOUR PLATE

In 2010 the United States Department of Agriculture (USDA) released a new nutrition education program called ChooseMyPlate. One of the ChooseMyPlate tips is to fill half your plate with fruits and vegetables. While many of the *Skinny-Size It* entrée recipes incorporate fruits and vegetables, it is still important to work toward filling at least half your plate with these foods. Check out the side dish recipes in the Deliciously Skinny Sides chapter (see recipes on pages 97–126) for great ways to work more vegetables into your meals. To add fruit to your meals, try pairing entrées with Applesauce (see recipe on page 149) or fresh-cut fruit, like apples, oranges, peaches or strawberries.

The average dinner plate has increased in size by about 23 percent since 1900. In the good old days, dinner plates were in the neighborhood of ten inches in diameter; however, today they are twelve inches in diameter or more. Try downsizing your dinner plate to help curb portion sizes, unless you are already filling it with *Skinny-Size It* dishes, in which case you are loading up on fruits and vegetables.

In addition, research has found that serving foods on a plate that creates a strong visual contrast can help you to keep better track of your portion size. For example, when serving pasta with red spaghetti sauce on a red plate, you could unwittingly enlarge the portion. Serving the same dish on a white plate would create a stronger visual contrast, enabling you to control the portion size better. The bottom line is that when choosing plate color, white is best in most cases as it creates the greatest visual contrast. When choosing plate size, there's no need to go as small as a coffee-cup saucer, but certainly steer clear of jumbo plates. And of course, when filling your plate, fill at least half of it with fruits and vegetables!

MEAT LOAF MUFFINS

Yield: 6 servings (2 muffins each)

Before:

Typically, meat loaf is made with higher-fat ground beef (around 80 percent lean and 20 percent fat), incorporates whole eggs and plain bread crumbs, and has minimal vegetables added. That combination results in a high calorie count and high total fat, saturated fat and sodium levels.

Skinny-Size It:

The combination of lean grass-fed beef, egg whites, ground flaxseed, more vegetables and whole-wheat panko bread crumbs skinnies up this recipe in a hurry. This meat loaf is full of flavor and has just 180 calories per serving, 6 grams of fat and 2 grams of saturated fat. Plus, grass-fed beef can have a healthier overall fat profile compared to conventional beef, with less saturated fat and more of the healthier unsaturated fat.

Ingredients

Nonstick cooking spray, for greasing the muffin tins

1 pound lean grass-fed ground beef

½ cup whole-wheat panko bread crumbs

½ cup shredded carrots

½ cup finely diced sweet onion

¼ cup beer (ale, lager or stout)

2 large egg whites, beaten

3 tablespoons ground flaxseed

¼ cup Maple BBQ Sauce (see recipe on page 156)

Directions

1. Preheat the oven to 350°F. Lightly coat the wells of a 12-cup muffin tin with cooking spray.

2. In a large mixing bowl, combine all the ingredients, except the Maple BBQ Sauce, and mix well.

3. Divide the meat loaf mixture into 12 portions and pack it into the wells of the prepared muffin tin.

4. Bake for 20 to 25 minutes, or until the meat loaf muffins are thoroughly cooked. (You can also press the meat loaf mixture into a 9 x 9-inch baking dish and bake for 30 minutes, or until thoroughly cooked.)

5. Arrange the meat loaf muffins on 6 individual plates, drizzle with the Maple BBQ Sauce, and serve at once.

Nutrition Facts (per serving)

180 calories, 6 grams fat, 2 grams saturated fat, 0 grams trans fat, 45 milligrams cholesterol, 170 milligrams sodium, 12 grams carbohydrates, 2 grams fiber, 5 grams sugar, 19 grams protein

BLACKENED SALMON WITH MANGO SALSA

Yield: 4 servings

Salmon all by itself is heart healthy as it is full of healthy fats.

Before:

Often salmon is served in large portions (8 ounces or more), which is about double the amount that most people need in one meal.

Skinny-Size It:

Decrease the salmon portion size to 4 ounces, which will still deliver 25 grams of protein and will make room for other healthy foods on the plate. Blackening the salmon with Cajun seasoning adds superb flavor, and topping it with a fresh mango salsa and plain nonfat Greek yogurt balances out the spice.

Skinny Tip:

Consuming fatty fish, such as wild salmon, mackerel, albacore tuna, sardines and herring, twice a week is healthy for your heart. For example, a 4-ounce serving of salmon has about 1.9 grams of omega-3 fatty acids, a healthy fat that has been linked to improved heart health and even to the prevention of some types of cancer (e.g., skin cancer).

Ingredients

1 tablespoon freshly squeezed lime juice

1 teaspoon honey

1 cup cubed mango

2 plum tomatoes, diced

½ cup diced sweet onion

1½ teaspoons minced fresh cilantro

1 pound wild salmon fillets (4 ounces each)

2 teaspoons Cajun seasoning

Nonstick cooking spray, for greasing the skillet

¼ cup plain nonfat Greek yogurt

Directions

1. In a medium-size mixing bowl, prepare the mango salsa by stirring together the lime juice and honey. Add the mango, tomatoes, onions and cilantro, and mix thoroughly. Set aside.
2. Prepare the salmon by rubbing one side of each fillet with the Cajun seasoning.
3. Lightly coat a large skillet with cooking spray and heat it over medium heat. Place the salmon fillets in a single layer in the skillet and cook until golden brown on one side, about 4 to 5 minutes, depending on the thickness of the fillets. Turn the fillets over with a spatula and cook until the other side is golden brown, about 4 to 5 minutes.
4. Arrange the salmon fillets on 4 individual plates and top with the mango salsa and the yogurt. Serve at once.

Nutrition Facts (per serving)

220 calories, 7 grams fat, 1 gram saturated fat, 0 grams trans fat, 60 milligrams cholesterol, 580 milligrams sodium, 13 grams carbohydrates, 2 grams fiber, 10 grams sugar, 25 grams protein

TRADITIONAL GENERAL TSO'S CHICKEN

Yield: 4 servings

Before:

During the 1970s, Taiwanese chefs introduced the Hunan dish General Tso's Chicken in the Hunan restaurants they had opened in New York City. The deep-fried chicken and the sweetened sauce of this dish appealed to the mainstream American palate. Depending on how it is prepared, a serving of General Tso's Chicken can have upwards of 700 calories and 20 grams of fat.

Skinny-Size It:

The Skinny-Size It version of General Tso's Chicken retains the original flavors without all the oil. The chicken is stir-fried rather than deep-fried, effectively cutting down the amount of fat and calories found in the original recipe. This version also features toasted cashews, which add crunch. A serving of this Traditional General Tso's Chicken, including the rice, contains only 460 calories and 11 grams of fat.

Ingredients

2 large egg whites

2 tablespoons cornstarch, plus 1 tablespoon for the sauce

2 tablespoons rice wine or dry sherry, plus 1 tablespoon for the sauce

1 tablespoon lite soy sauce, plus 1 tablespoon for the sauce

1 pound boneless, skinless chicken breast, cut into 1-inch cubes

1 tablespoon low-sodium chicken broth, plus 3 tablespoons for the sauce

2 teaspoons white vinegar

2 teaspoons sugar

2 ounces (½ cup) cashews

1 teaspoon sesame oil

3 small dried red chili peppers (or more,
    if desired)

½ cup thinly sliced scallions

2 tablespoons minced garlic

2 tablespoons minced fresh ginger

4 cups steamed broccoli

2 cups cooked brown rice

Directions

1. In a medium-size mixing bowl, whisk together
   the egg whites, 2 tablespoons of the cornstarch,
   2 tablespoons of the rice wine or dry sherry and
   1 tablespoon of the soy sauce. Add the chicken to
   the marinade and toss to coat. Cover and marinate
   in the refrigerator for 2 to 4 hours (or overnight).

2. In a small mixing bowl, prepare the sauce by
   combining the remaining 1 tablespoon cornstarch and
   1 tablespoon of the chicken stock, and whisk together
   until smooth. Add the remaining 3 tablespoons
   chicken stock, the remaining 1 tablespoon rice
   wine or dry sherry, the remaining 1 tablespoon soy
   sauce, the vinegar and sugar, and whisk to combine.
   Set the sauce aside.

3. Cook the cashews in a dry wok over medium heat
   until they are lightly toasted, about 1 to 2 minutes.
   Remove the cashews to a small bowl and set aside.

4. Heat the sesame oil in the wok over medium heat. Remove the chicken cubes from the marinade with a slotted spoon and slide them gently into the hot oil, using the sides of the wok to minimize splashing. (Caution! Even though there is a small amount of oil in the wok, it can splash if you drop the chicken in too quickly. Unfortunately, I know from experience.) Stir-fry the chicken for about 3 or 4 minutes, or until cooked thoroughly. Then remove the chicken to a clean medium-size bowl and set aside. Discard the leftover marinade.

5. Add the dried chili peppers to the wok and stir-fry until lightly browned, about 1 minute. Then add the scallions, garlic and ginger, and stir-fry for 30 seconds to 1 minute. Add the reserved sauce to the wok, bring it to a boil and cook until it thickens, about 1 to 2 minutes. Add the reserved chicken to the wok and stir to coat with the sauce.

6. Spoon the rice onto 4 individual plates or into bowls and top with the steamed broccoli and the stir-fried chicken. Garnish with the toasted cashews, and serve at once.

Nutrition Facts (per serving)

460 calories, 11 grams fat, 2 grams saturated fat, 0 grams trans fat, 65 milligrams cholesterol, 580 milligrams sodium, 49 grams carbohydrates, 5 grams fiber, 5 grams sugar, 39 grams protein

CRUNCHY TACOS

Yield: 4 servings (2 tacos each)

Before:

One small crunchy taco from a Mexican restaurant can have 170 calories or more, 10 grams of fat or more and only 3 grams of fiber, and you will likely order more than one small crunchy taco.

Skinny-Size It:

Selecting a crunchy taco shell made from whole-grain corn is a perfect way to start making your own crunchy tacos. Then add some Southwestern flair by swapping the traditional beef filling for *calabacitas,* a sautéed medley of beans, yellow squash, zucchini, red and green peppers, corn and seasoning (see recipe on page 123). Next, top the tacos with reduced-fat cheese and plain nonfat yogurt in place of sour cream, while adding healthy fats with the Salsa-Mole (mashed avocados and salsa; see recipe on page 146). The result is a serving of two tacos with only 14 grams of fat, and with 12 grams of fiber.

Skinny Shopping:

A must buy when it comes to crunchy taco shells, whole-grain corn taco shells have only 110 calories per two-shell serving, but the best part is they contain 5 grams of fiber!

Ingredients

1⅓ cups Salsa-Mole (see recipe on page 146)

2 plum tomatoes, diced

½ small sweet onion, peeled and diced

½ large red bell pepper, seeded, deribbed and diced

¼ medium cucumber, chopped

2 ounces light cheddar cheese, shredded

¼ cup plain nonfat Greek yogurt

¼ cup sliced black olives

8 crunchy whole-grain taco shells

2 cups Calabacitas (see recipe on page 123)

Directions

1. Place the Salsa-Mole, tomatoes, onions, peppers, cucumbers, cheese, yogurt and black olives in individual serving bowls.
2. Arrange 2 taco shells on each of 4 individual plates and fill each shell with the Calabacitas. Have everyone at the table assemble their own tacos, adding the toppings of their choice.

Nutrition Facts (per serving)

300 calories, 14 grams fat, 2.5 grams saturated fat, 0 grams trans fat, 5 milligrams cholesterol, 510 milligrams sodium, 38 grams carbohydrates, 12 grams fiber, 6 grams sugar, 13 grams protein

BUTTERNUT SOBA NOODLE BOWL

Yield: 4 servings

Before:

Many Asian-flavored dishes have a lot of added oil, which drives up the calories and the fat content of the dish, and are loaded with sodium.

Skinny-Size It:

Sesame oil is so rich tasting that a little goes a long way, and so it's easy to cut the fat and up the flavor of a dish at the same time. Making your own Honey-Sesame Soy Sauce (see recipe on page 152) is an excellent way to trim the fat, sodium and sugar content of a dish, as well.

Skinny Shopping:

Soba noodles are typically found in the ethnic food section of the grocery store. They are traditionally a noodle made with 100 percent buckwheat flour. Many varieties are a blend of wheat and buckwheat flours, which is still nutritionally a great choice although the flavor and texture will be lighter compared to soba noodle varieties made with 100 percent buckwheat flour.

Ingredients

1 medium butternut squash, cut in half, seeded and baked until tender

1 tablespoon sesame oil

One 8-ounce package soba (buckwheat)
noodles, cooked

¼ cup Honey-Sesame Soy Sauce (see recipe
on page 152)

Directions

1. Once the baked butternut squash is cool enough
   to handle, remove the skin and cut the flesh into
   ½-inch cubes.
2. Heat the sesame oil in a wok over medium heat.
   Slide the squash cubes gently into the hot oil,
   using the sides of the wok to minimize splashing,
   and stir-fry for about 2 to 3 minutes.
3. Add the cooked soba noodles and the Honey-Sesame
   Soy Sauce, and stir to coat the squash and the noodles.
   Serve at once.

Nutrition Facts (per serving)

340 calories, 7 grams fat, 1 gram saturated fat, 0 grams trans
fat, 0 milligrams cholesterol, 410 milligrams sodium, 64 grams
carbohydrates, 2 grams fiber, 10 grams sugar, 11 grams protein

CHICKEN PAD THAI

Yield: 4 servings

Before:

Pad thai can surpass 700 calories per serving and have a teaspoon's worth of sodium (2,300 milligrams), which is more
than some people should have in an entire day.

Skinny-Size It:

Make your own pad thai sauce to cut down on the sodium, swapping lite soy sauce for regular soy sauce and adding lots of fresh flavor from garlic and gingerroot. This recipe boasts a cup of veggies and half a cup of soba noodles per serving, boosting the fiber and providing longer-lasting energy.

Ingredients

1 tablespoon lite soy sauce

1 tablespoon creamy natural peanut butter

1 tablespoon water

1 teaspoon chili paste

3 tablespoons extra-virgin olive oil

1 teaspoon minced garlic

1 teaspoon minced gingerroot

4 cups chopped vegetables (broccoli, carrots, snap peas), steamed

8 ounces boneless, skinless chicken breast, cut into 1-inch pieces

2 cups cooked soba (buckwheat) noodles

1 tablespoon brown sugar

1 tablespoon apple cider vinegar

Directions

1. In a small mixing bowl, whisk together the soy sauce, peanut butter, water and chili paste until smooth. Set the sauce aside.

2. Heat the olive oil in a wok or a large skillet over medium-high heat. When the oil is hot, add the garlic and ginger and cook, stirring frequently, until fragrant, about 1 minute.

3. Slide the steamed vegetables and the chicken gently into the hot oil, using the sides of the wok to minimize splashing, and stir-fry until the chicken has browned and is cooked through, about 2 minutes. Then add the cooked noodles.

4. Stir in the reserved sauce, the brown sugar and vinegar, and toss the contents of the wok to coat. Cook until the noodles are heated through, about 2 minutes. Serve at once.

Nutrition Facts (per serving)

360 calories, 16 grams fat, 2.5 grams saturated fat, 0 grams trans fat, 50 milligrams cholesterol, 280 milligrams sodium, 30 grams carbohydrates, 4 grams fiber, 6 grams sugar, 26 grams protein

VEGGIE PAELLA

Yield: 6 servings

Before:

Paella, a traditional rice dish that originated on the East Coast of Spain, typically showcases high-fat meats, such as sausage.

Skinny Shopping:

Always keep frozen butternut squash cubes (and other frozen veggies, too) on hand, as they are a great addition to many dishes and a perfect, simple side dish.

Skinny-Size It:

Incorporate plenty of vegetables in place of the meat, and it won't even be missed. All the veggies and the brown rice in this recipe result in 7 grams of fiber per serving and provide immune-boosting vitamin A and vitamin C.

Ingredients

1 teaspoon extra-virgin olive oil

2 cloves garlic, peeled and minced

1 teaspoon garlic powder

2 cups frozen butternut squash cubes

2 cups frozen green beans

One 14-ounce can diced tomatoes

1 medium yellow squash, ends cut off and cut into bite-size pieces (1 cup)

1 medium zucchini, ends cut off and cut into bite-size pieces (1 cup)

2 medium carrots, peeled and diced (1 cup)

1 cup asparagus, cut into bite-size pieces

$\frac{1}{2}$ teaspoon paprika

$\frac{1}{8}$ teaspoon ground allspice

3 cups cooked brown rice

1 cup low-sodium vegetable broth

Sea salt and freshly ground black pepper, to taste

Directions

1. Heat the olive oil in a Dutch oven or a large pot over medium heat. Sauté the garlic and garlic powder until just fragrant, about 1 minute.

2. Add the butternut squash, green beans, tomatoes, yellow squash, zucchini, carrots, asparagus, paprika and allspice. Simmer for 10 minutes.

3. Add the cooked rice and vegetable broth, and cook for 10 minutes more, or until the liquid is absorbed. Season with sea salt and pepper, and serve at once.

Nutrition Facts (per serving)

200 calories, 2 grams fat, 0 grams saturated fat, 0 grams trans fat, 0 milligrams cholesterol, 310 milligrams sodium, 42 grams carbohydrates, 7 grams fiber, 7 grams sugar, 6 grams protein

CHEESY CHICKEN

Yield: 4 servings

Before:

Usually the word *cheesy* in a recipe is a red flag, because it commonly indicates that a dish has a heavy, creamy cheese sauce. One cheesy dish could potentially contain as much fat (or more) as you need in an entire day.

Skinny-Size It:

The cheese sauce in Cheesy Chicken has fresh vegetables as a foundation, and they add volume and fiber without contributing excess calories. Additionally, the sauce is made with fat-free half-and-half (another exception to my skip fat-free dairy suggestion), which is an excellent ingredient for thickening a sauce without adding fat. Finally, a light cheddar cheese lends the cheesy texture and flavor without sending the dish over the calorie cliff. Cheesy Chicken contains a grand total of 160 calories and 4.5 grams of fat per serving.

Ingredients

2 plum tomatoes, diced

1 medium sweet onion, peeled and diced

2 cloves garlic, peeled and minced

2 boneless, skinless chicken breasts, sliced
(about 4 ounces each)

1 tablespoon all-purpose white flour

½ cup fat-free half-and-half

2 ounces shredded light cheddar cheese
(such as Cabot Sharp Light Cheddar Cheese)

Directions

1. In a large skillet over medium heat, sauté the tomatoes
   and onions until tender, about 5 to 7 minutes. Add
   the garlic and sauté 1 minute more.
2. Add the chicken and sauté for 10 to 15 minutes,
   or until it is cooked through.
3. Stir in the flour and then the half-and-half. Bring to
   a boil, stirring frequently, and allow it to bubble for
   1 minute to thicken the sauce.
4. Add the cheese and stir until it has melted.
5. Serving Suggestion: Serve over brown rice or with fresh
   steamed vegetables, such as broccoli or asparagus.

Nutrition Facts (per serving
without the rice or the vegetables)

160 calories, 4.5 grams fat, 2 grams saturated fat, 0 grams trans
fat, 45 milligrams cholesterol, 160 milligrams sodium, 11 grams
carbohydrates, 1 gram fiber, 5 grams sugar, 19 grams protein

PAN-SEARED TUNA

Yield: 4 servings

Before:

Pan-seared tuna recipes sometimes call for as much as 2 tablespoons of oil per 6 ounces of tuna, which adds about 20 grams of fat and 180 calories to the serving.

Skinny-Size It:

Pan searing tuna the Skinny way requires a hot skillet and a light coating of cooking spray. When prepared the Skinny way, a 4-ounce tuna fillet has 160 calories and 6 grams of total fat, and provides 1.5 grams of polyunsaturated fat, some of which is omega-3 fatty acids, which are known to help heart health. Plus this dish tops the tuna with Avocado Salsa (see recipe on page 161), which has belly slimming mono-unsaturated fat.

Ingredients

Nonstick cooking spray, for greasing the skillet

1 pound wild-caught tuna fillets (4 ounces each)

Freshly cracked black pepper, to taste

½ cup Avocado Salsa (see recipe on page 161)

Directions

1. Lightly coat a large skillet with cooking spray and heat over medium heat.
2. Season the tuna fillets with pepper. Arrange the fillets in the skillet and sear on each side for 1 to 2 minutes.
3. Serve the pan-seared tuna at once with the Avocado Salsa.

Nutrition Facts (per serving)

240 calories, 12 grams fat, 2.5 grams saturated fat, 0 grams trans fat, 45 milligrams cholesterol, 120 milligrams sodium, 6 grams carbohydrates, 3 grams fiber, < 1 gram sugar, 28 grams protein

VEGGIE POTPIE

Yield: 6 servings

Potpie in a Skinny cookbook? You bet! This potpie is loaded with veggies and is absolutely delicious.

Before:

Many store-bought potpies and homemade potpies have 400 or more calories per serving and upwards of 25 grams of fat.

Skinny Tip:

Nutritional yeast is used in a lot of vegan recipes because it is fortified with B vitamins and adds flavor. It is an excellent addition to the gravy in this potpie. You can find nutritional yeast in the baking aisle or the natural food section of your grocery store.

Skinny-Size It:

When you load the potpie up with veggies and use a flavorful sauce, you eliminate half the calories and fat. So go ahead and enjoy all the comforts of potpie, a perfect meal on a cold winter's night! I love the memory from the night when my dad and my brother were over for dinner and this recipe. After they started eating, I told them that the "gravy" wasn't really gravy at all, but rather a delicious sauce, and to my delight, they liked the taste so much that they both went back for second helpings!

Ingredients

2 cups cubed sweet potatoes

2 cups sliced carrots

2 cups cubed butternut squash

3 teaspoons extra-virgin olive oil

One 8-ounce package firm tofu, drained and cubed

1 sliced medium sweet onion

4 cloves garlic, peeled and minced

1⅓ cups water

½ cup nutritional yeast

¼ cup all-purpose white flour

2 tablespoons lite soy sauce

1 teaspoon onion powder

1 teaspoon garlic powder

½ teaspoon sea salt

One 9-inch pie crust

Directions

1. Preheat the oven to 350°F.
2. Combine the sweet potatoes, carrots and butternut squash in a Dutch oven or a large soup pot, cover with water, and bring the water to a boil over medium-high heat. Once it boils, reduce the heat

to medium and cook the vegetables until tender, about 10 minutes. Drain the vegetables and set aside.

3. Heat the olive oil in a large skillet over medium heat, and sauté the tofu, onions and garlic until the onions are tender, about 5 to 7 minutes. Add the sautéed tofu, onions and garlic to the reserved boiled vegetables.

4. Heat the water, nutritional yeast, flour, soy sauce, onion powder, garlic powder and sea salt in a medium-size soup pot over medium heat, and cook, stirring constantly, until thickened, about 7 to 9 minutes. Add half the sauce to the reserved vegetable-tofu mixture.

5. Arrange the pie crust in a 9-inch pie dish. Fill the pie crust with the reserved vegetable-tofu mixture. Spoon the remaining sauce over the pie filling.

6. Bake the potpie until the crust is golden brown and the filling is bubbly, about 1 hour.

Nutrition Facts (per serving)

290 calories, 12 grams fat, 3 grams saturated fat, 0 grams trans fat, < 5 milligrams cholesterol, 590 milligrams sodium, 37 grams carbohydrates, 6 grams fiber, 6 grams sugar, 11 grams protein

PEACHY GINGER CHICKEN

Yield: 4 servings

Before:

The original version of this recipe calls for half a cup of feta cheese and half a cup of olive oil (in the dressing), for a total of about 370 calories and 22 grams of fat per serving.

Skinny-Size It:

Skimping on the feta cheese doesn't diminish the feta flavor and creamy texture, but it does cut the fat. Revamping the dressing by replacing some of the oil with white vinegar lowers the calories and fat. The sautéed spinach and grilled peaches add fiber and fresh flavors to the recipe, while keeping the dish at 250 calories and 9 grams of fat per serving.

Ingredients

Dressing

¼ cup extra-virgin olive oil

¼ cup white vinegar

2 tablespoons dry sherry

1 tablespoon agave nectar

2 teaspoons ground ginger

1 teaspoon dried thyme

½ teaspoon crushed red pepper (optional)

Peachy Chicken

4 boneless, skinless chicken breasts
   (about 4 ounces each)

2 medium peaches, halved and pitted

4 cups baby spinach

¼ cup crumbled feta cheese

Directions

1. In a medium-size bowl, prepare the dressing by whisking all the dressing ingredients together or by combining them in a salad dressing shaker and shaking vigorously. Set aside 1 tablespoon of the dressing and brush over the chicken. Let the chicken stand in the refrigerator for 15 minutes.

2. Preheat the grill to medium-high. Grill the chicken, turning occasionally, until cooked thoroughly, about 15 minutes. Remove the chicken to a large plate.

3. Place the peaches, cut side down, on the grill and cook for 5 minutes. Remove the peaches to a small plate.

4. Cut the grilled chicken and peaches into 1-inch slices.

5. In a large skillet, sauté the spinach with 1 tablespoon of the reserved dressing over medium heat until the spinach is wilted, about 2 to 3 minutes.

6. Arrange the sautéed spinach on 4 individual serving plates and top with the grilled chicken and peach slices. Garnish with the feta cheese and the remaining dressing, and serve at once.

Nutrition Facts (per serving)

250 calories, 9 grams fat, 2.5 grams saturated fat, 0 grams trans fat, 75 milligrams cholesterol, 260 milligrams sodium, 10 grams carbohydrates, 1 gram fiber, 7 grams sugar, 29 grams protein

SWEET POTATO NOODLE BOWL

Yield: 4 servings

Before:

Pasta dishes are notorious for being loaded with calories and low-quality carbohydrates.

Skinny-Size It:

Swap traditional noodles for soba (buckwheat) noodles and add plenty of colorful vegetables to bring down the calorie count per serving. The colorful vegetables in this dish supply a healthy dose of your daily vitamin and mineral needs. Each serving provides 310 percent of the daily value for vitamin A, 120 percent of the daily value for vitamin C, 15 percent of the daily value for calcium and 20 percent of the daily value for iron.

Ingredients

One 8-ounce package soba (buckwheat) noodles

1 teaspoon extra-virgin olive oil

3 cloves garlic, peeled and minced

3 cups shredded sweet potato

1 cup finely diced red bell pepper

2 ounces feta cheese, crumbled

Directions

1. Prepare the soba noodles according to the package instructions. Drain, reserving ½ cup of the noodle water.
2. Heat the olive oil in a large skillet and sauté the garlic until just fragrant, about 1 minute.

3. Add the sweet potatoes, peppers and reserved noodle water, and cook for 5 to 7 minutes. Cover the skillet, lower the heat to medium-low and simmer the vegetables until they are tender, about 3 to 5 minutes.
4. In a large serving bowl, combine the cooked soba noodles and the veggie mixture.
5. Serve in individual bowls, garnished with feta cheese.

Nutrition Facts (per serving)

350 calories, 6 grams fat, 2.5 grams saturated fat, 0 grams trans fat, 15 milligrams cholesterol, 330 milligrams sodium, 63 grams carbohydrates, 6 grams fiber, 9 grams sugar, 12 grams protein

POLENTA LASAGNA

Yield: 6 servings

Before:

Traditional lasagna is filled with large amounts of cheese, including ricotta, Parmesan and mozzarella. Ground beef or sausage are often key ingredients in lasagnas, which can make the calories and fat pile up in a hurry. In fact, restaurant versions of lasagna can have 900 calories and 50 grams of fat or more per serving.

Skinny-Size It:

When lasagna is made with roasted vegetables, homemade tomato sauce and a modest amount of mozzarella cheese, the calorie count drops precipitously. A serving of Polenta Lasagna has just 260 calories and 7 grams of fat.

Ingredients

Polenta

4 cups water

1 1/4 cups coarse ground yellow cornmeal

1/4 teaspoon minced fresh rosemary

Filling

1 large eggplant

2 cups diced fresh mushrooms (portabella, shiitake or button)

1 cup diced sweet onion

2 cloves garlic, peeled and minced

1/4 cup water

One 16-ounce jar roasted red peppers, drained and cut into 1/2-inch pieces

4 ounces part-skim mozzarella cheese, shredded

2 tablespoons minced fresh basil

2 tablespoons fresh oregano

3 cups Garlic Tomato Spaghetti Sauce (see recipe on page 165) or store-bought spaghetti sauce

Directions

1. Prepare the polenta by bringing the water to a boil in a large saucepan over medium-high heat. Gradually whisk in the cornmeal and cook, whisking, until it is thick, 10 to 15 minutes. Whisk in the rosemary.

2. Spoon the polenta into two 9 x 9-inch baking pans and spread it evenly with a spoon. The polenta will be about 3/4 inch thick. Cover the polenta and place it in the refrigerator.

3. Preheat the oven to 425°F.

4. Prepare the eggplant by piercing it several times with a fork and then placing it in a baking dish or on a baking sheet. Roast the eggplant for 45 minutes, or until the flesh is soft and the skin is charred. Let the eggplant cool slightly, remove the charred skin and then cut it into bite-size pieces and set aside.

5. To make the vegetable filling, combine the mushrooms, onions, garlic and water in a large skillet and cook over medium heat until the liquid evaporates. Transfer the mushroom-onion mixture to a large mixing bowl and stir in the reserved eggplant, peppers, half the mozzarella, basil and oregano.

6. Pour 1 cup of the spaghetti sauce into a 9 x 13-inch baking dish and spread it around so that the bottom is coated evenly. Then place half the reserved polenta atop the tomato sauce in an even layer, cutting it into strips if necessary. Next, spoon the vegetable filling evenly over the polenta and then top the filling with the remaining polenta in an even layer. Spoon the remaining 2 cups spaghetti sauce atop the polenta and then sprinkle the remaining mozzarella over the top.

7. Bake for 30 minutes, or until the lasagna is heated through and the cheese has melted. Serve at once.

Nutrition Facts (per serving)

260 calories, 7 grams fat, 2.5 grams saturated fat, 0 grams trans fat, 10 milligrams cholesterol, 370 milligrams sodium, 43 grams carbohydrates, 9 grams fiber, 10 grams sugar, 11 grams protein

EGGPLANT MOZZARELLA

Yield: 6 servings

Before:

Eggplant Parmesan ordered at a restaurant sometimes arrives at the table in a pool of oil.

Skinny-Size It:

This Skinny-Size It version of the traditionally calorie-laden dish has only 160 calories and 4 grams of fat per serving, as well as 6 grams of fiber. One key ingredient is whole-wheat panko bread crumbs, which help boost the fiber content and give the dish its crispiness—without frying.

Skinny Skip:

Oil can be omitted altogether in many dishes, and when fresh flavors are maximized, the excess fat won't even be missed. Eggplant Parmesan is a prime example of how you can slim down a traditionally oily dish without even missing the fat. In fact, the revamped version has become a regular with my family because we all, the little guys included, love this dish!

Ingredients

1 medium eggplant

½ teaspoon sea salt

1 cup whole-wheat panko bread crumbs

1 tablespoon garlic powder

1 tablespoon oregano

1 cup low-fat milk plus 1 tablespoon white vinegar
(buttermilk)

2 cups Garlic Tomato Spaghetti Sauce
(see recipe on page 165)

½ cup shredded part-skim mozzarella cheese

Directions

1. Cut the eggplant into ¼-inch slices. Arrange
   the eggplant slices on a baking sheet and sprinkle
   with the sea salt. Let the eggplant sit for 30 minutes
   to remove the bitterness. Then pat with a paper
   towel to absorb the liquid and remove the salt. Rinse
   the eggplant under cold water to remove any excess
   salt, if desired.

2. Preheat the oven to 425°F.

3. Combine the bread crumbs with the garlic powder
   and oregano. Pour the bread crumb mixture and the
   buttermilk into individual shallow bowls.

4. Dip an eggplant slice into the buttermilk and then into
   the bread crumbs to coat. Then place it on a 9 x 13-inch
   baking sheet. Repeat until all the eggplant slices have
   been breaded.

5. Bake the eggplant slices for 25 to 30 minutes, or until
   tender and lightly browned, turning once during bake
   time. After baking, reduce the oven temperature
   to 350°F.

6. Pour ½ cup of the spaghetti sauce into a 9 x 9-inch
   baking dish and spread it around so that the bottom
   is coated evenly. Place some of the breaded eggplant
   slices atop the sauce, forming an even single layer, and
   then spoon ½ cup of the spaghetti sauce over the

eggplant. Layer the remaining eggplant slices atop the sauce. Spoon the remaining 1 cup spaghetti sauce atop the eggplant and then sprinkle the mozzarella over the top.

7. Bake the Eggplant Mozzarella for 20 minutes, or until the cheese is melted and the sauce is heated through. Serve at once.

Nutrition Facts (per serving)

160 calories, 4 grams fat, 1.5 grams saturated fat, 0 grams trans fat, 5 milligrams cholesterol, 190 milligrams sodium, 24 grams carbohydrates, 6 grams fiber, 6 grams sugar, 8 grams protein

PASTA WITH SEAFOOD AND VODKA CREAM SAUCE

Yield: 6 servings

Before:

Generally, I would not recommend traditionally prepared cream sauce dishes as a Skinny choice!

Skinny Swap:

Most cream sauces are made with heavy cream. However, this *Skinny-Size-It* recipe is made with unsweetened almond milk and gains its flavor from the fresh garlic, the roasted red peppers and other vegetables, and the crab or lobster.

Skinny-Size It:

When the base of the cream sauce is prepared with minimal added fat, it moves cream sauce dishes from the caution zone to go for it! Each serving of this pasta dish has 330 calories, 9 grams of fat and 7 grams of belly-filling fiber.

Ingredients

1½ tablespoons unsalted margarine or butter

2 tablespoons all-purpose white flour

3 cloves garlic, peeled and minced

2 cups unsweetened almond milk or low-fat milk

1 cup roasted red peppers, pureed

1 ounce vodka

1 cup broccoli, cooked and cut into bite-size pieces

1 cup asparagus, cooked and cut into bite-size pieces

½ cup sliced black olives

1 cup flaked crab meat or diced lobster meat

2 cups baby spinach

2 cups cooked whole-wheat pasta or
    brown-rice pasta

Directions

1. Melt the margarine in a large saucepan over medium-low heat. Whisk in the flour and then add the garlic and cook for 1 minute. Add the milk and bring it to a boil, stirring frequently. Allow the sauce to bubble for 1 minute more.

2. Add the peppers and vodka to the sauce and stir well. Then add the broccoli, asparagus and black olives, and cook for 10 minutes. Gently fold in the crab or lobster and cook for 3 minutes more.

3. Arrange the spinach at the bottom of 6 individual serving bowls, top with the pasta and then the seafood-vegetable mixture, and serve at once.

Nutrition Facts (per serving)

330 calories, 9 grams fat, 3 grams saturated fat, 0 grams trans fat, 60 milligrams cholesterol, 410 milligrams sodium, 32 grams carbohydrates, 7 grams fiber, 2 grams sugar, 23 grams protein

4

....

Deliciously Skinny Sides

Filling your plate at least half full with fruits and vegetables will get easier with these side dish recipes! Another quarter of your plate should be dedicated to grains, and all the grain-based recipes in *Skinny-Size It* feature whole grains. As I mentioned earlier, although the USDA's recommended daily goal is to make half your grains whole grains, the Skinny-Size It recommendation is to make almost all your grains whole grains.

If you or those for whom you cook need to consume more vegetables and fruit, try leaving the fruit and vegetable dishes that you are serving with the meal at the table to easily allow for seconds! Also, serve the foods you should be eating more of in larger bowls. Research shows that people serve themselves more when serving dishes are larger and, consequently, eat more. In fact, one study found that when served a large bowl of food with a large utensil, participants ate 56 percent more compared to when they were served the same food in a smaller bowl. Of course, when it comes to potato chips, this is not good news. However, when we are talking about fruits and vegetables, selecting larger dishware may help to increase the amount you eat and in turn help fill you up on lower-calorie dishes.

BALSAMIC BRUSSELS WITH BACON

Yield: 4 servings

Before:
Some Brussels sprouts with bacon recipes contain far too much bacon, and many have added oil, as well.

Skinny-Size It:
This Skinny version brings in flavor with balsamic vinegar, gets a little sweetness from agave nectar and contains a scant amount of oil. The mere two slices of bacon impart lots of flavor to this dish, while keeping the calories and fat content under control. A single serving has only 4 grams of fat.

Ingredients

¼ cup balsamic vinegar

2 teaspoons agave nectar

2 teaspoons extra-virgin olive oil

1 pound of Brussels sprouts, trimmed and halved (about 3 cups)

2 slices cooked center-cut bacon, crumbled

Directions

1. Preheat the oven to 350°F.
2. In a large bowl, mix together the vinegar, agave nectar and olive oil. Add the Brussels sprouts and stir to coat.
3. Transfer the Brussels sprouts to a baking dish and roast for 25 to 30 minutes, or until they are tender. Transfer them to a serving dish, garnish with the crumbled bacon, and serve at once.

Nutrition Facts (per serving)

90 calories, 4 grams fat, 1 gram saturated fat, 0 grams trans fat, < 5 milligrams cholesterol, 65 milligrams sodium, 11 grams carbohydrates, 3 grams fiber, 4 grams sugar, 4 grams protein

ROASTED SUMMER VEGETABLES

Yield: 4 servings

Before:

Roasted vegetable dishes tend to be heavy due to the amount of added oil or butter. Every tablespoon of olive oil added to a dish translates into 120 calories and 14 grams of fat, and although olive oil is a healthy unsaturated fat, it still kicks up the calorie and fat content of a recipe.

Skinny-Size It:

Roast a medley of summer vegetables, such as yellow squash, zucchini, peppers and onions, with a small amount of olive oil and garlic to create a dish that has lots of flavor and only 70 calories per serving.

Ingredients

1 medium yellow squash, ends cut off, halved lengthwise and cut into ¼-inch half-moons

1 medium zucchini, ends cut off, halved lengthwise and cut into ¼-inch half-moons

1 medium red bell pepper, seeded, deribbed and cut into 1-inch pieces

1 medium sweet onion, peeled and cut into ½-inch slices

4 cloves garlic, peeled and minced

1 tablespoon extra-virgin olive oil

Sea salt and freshly ground black pepper, to taste

Directions

1. Preheat the oven to 400°F.
2. Place the yellow squash, zucchini, peppers and onions on a baking sheet, add the garlic and olive oil, and toss to coat.
3. Bake the vegetables, stirring occasionally, until they are tender, about 35 to 40 minutes.
4. Season the roasted vegetables with sea salt and pepper, and serve at once.

Nutrition Facts (per serving)

70 calories, 3.5 grams fat, 0.5 grams saturated fat, 0 grams trans fat, 10 milligrams cholesterol, 10 milligrams sodium, 10 grams carbohydrates, 2 grams fiber, 5 grams sugar, 2 grams protein

SUN-DRIED TOMATO MORNAY SAUCE WITH STEAMED BROCCOLI

Yield: 4 servings

Before:

Mornay sauce is typically a béchamel sauce, made with whole milk, to which a combination of cheeses, traditionally Parmesan and Gruyère, is added. While it traditionally adorns seafood or vegetables, which are naturally lower in calories, this sauce will send you into the red zone pretty quickly, thanks to its fat content.

Skinny-Size It:

Creating a Skinny béchamel sauce with low-fat milk gets this Mornay sauce off to a great start! (You can't remove all the fat from the béchamel sauce, because some butter and flour are needed to thicken it.) Adding sun-dried tomatoes and a modest amount of Parmesan gives the Mornay sauce a wonderful taste, so you will not even miss the Gruyère. These swaps result in a savings of 100 calories and 8 grams of fat per serving.

Ingredients

1½ tablespoons unsalted butter

2 tablespoons all-purpose white flour

2 cups low-fat milk

1 ounce grated Parmesan cheese (¼ cup)

3 ounces thinly sliced dry-packed sun-dried tomatoes, soaked in warm water until soft and then drained (not oil-packed)

4 cups steamed broccoli

Directions

1. Melt the butter in a medium saucepan over medium-low heat. Stir in the flour and mix well, and then add the milk and whisk. Bring the mixture to a boil, whisking frequently to make a smooth sauce, and then let it bubble 1 minute more so it thickens.

2. Stir in the cheese and sun-dried tomatoes, and cook until the cheese is incorporated, about 1 minute.

3. Pour the sauce over the steamed broccoli, and serve at once.

Nutrition Facts (per serving)

170 calories, 8 grams fat, 4.5 grams saturated fat, 0 grams trans fat, 20 milligrams cholesterol, 310 milligrams sodium, 19 grams carbohydrates, 3 grams fiber, 4 grams sugar, 10 grams protein

MIXED VEGETABLE POLENTA

Yield: 8 servings

Before:

Polenta is essentially a light dish to which cheese and butter are often added for flavor.

Skinny-Size It:

My husband came up with this recipe and we like it so much that we even have it as a main dish. One key is switching from butter to nutrient-rich extra-virgin olive oil, and adding garlic powder for flavor, as well as plenty of mixed vegetables, results in a dish that is hearty enough to be served

as a main dish and simple enough to complement an entrée.
A single side dish serving has just 130 calories.

Ingredients

6 cups water

1 $3/4$ cups coarse ground yellow cornmeal

2 tablespoons extra-virgin olive oil

2 teaspoons garlic powder

$1/2$ teaspoon sea salt

One 10-ounce package frozen mixed vegetables,
cooked and drained

Directions

1. Prepare the polenta by bringing the water to a
   boil in a large saucepan over medium-high heat.
   Gradually whisk in the cornmeal and then add the
   olive oil, garlic powder and sea salt. Cook, whisking,
   until the polenta starts to thicken, 10 to 15 minutes.
   Then cook until the polenta has thickened, about
   15 minutes more.
2. Stir in the cooked mixed vegetables, and serve
   at once.

Nutrition Facts (per serving)

130 calories, 4 grams fat, 0 grams saturated fat, 0 grams trans
fat, 0 milligrams cholesterol, 160 milligrams sodium, 22 grams
carbohydrates, 3 grams fiber, 1 gram sugar, 3 grams protein

BUTTERMILK SCONES

Yield: 8 servings (1 scone each)

Before:

Most scones are made with strictly all-purpose white flour, and a batch can have as much as a whole stick of butter in it.

Skinny-Size It:

Make the Skinny swap of half the all-purpose white flour for whole-wheat flour to add fiber, vitamins and minerals to the scones. Then skimp on the amount of butter added, which still allows for a soft, flaky texture without all the added fat. The swaps and skimps result in a savings of 4 grams of fat per scone and the addition of 2 grams of fiber per scone.

Ingredients

Nonstick cooking spray, for greasing
   the baking sheet

1½ cups all-purpose white flour

1½ cups whole-wheat flour

2 tablespoons baking powder

¼ teaspoon sea salt

⅓ cup melted unsalted butter

1¼ cups low-fat milk plus 1 tablespoon white
   vinegar (buttermilk)

Directions

1. Preheat the oven to 425°F. Coat a baking sheet with cooking spray.

2. In a large mixing bowl, sift together the all-purpose white flour, the whole-wheat flour, baking powder and

sea salt. Add the melted butter and combine until the mixture resembles a coarse meal.

3. Add the buttermilk and mix until a soft dough forms.

4. Turn the dough out onto a lightly floured surface and shape it into a rectangle about $3/4$-inch thick and 4 inches wide. Cut the dough into 8 triangles of equal size and arrange them on the prepared baking sheet.

5. Bake for 10 to 15 minutes, or until the scones are lightly browned.

Nutrition Facts (per serving)

240 calories, 8 grams fat, 5 grams saturated fat, 0 grams trans fat, 20 milligrams cholesterol, 450 milligrams sodium, 36 grams carbohydrates, 3 grams fiber, 3 grams sugar, 7 grams protein

BBQ BLACK BEANS

Yield: 8 servings

Before:

Some traditional baked bean recipes and canned baked beans have 500 or more milligrams of sodium and upwards of 6 teaspoons of sugar (or around 24 grams of sugar) per serving.

Skinny-Size It:

Introducing plenty of onions and tomatoes for flavor, cutting out oil and reducing the amount of barbecue sauce results in a rejuvenated dish with a third the sugar compared to store-bought baked beans and 0 grams of fat.

Nutritional Powerhouse:

Onions are powerful heart disease and cancer fighters, thanks to their high concentration of allyl sulfides, and they are an excellent source of belly-helping inulin, vitamin C, fiber, folate and manganese. In this dish, the sweet onions and tomatoes are a perfect start, adding fresh flavor and reducing the amount of barbecue sauce needed.

Ingredients

3 medium tomatoes, diced

1 medium sweet onion, peeled and diced

2 cloves garlic, peeled and minced

3 cups cooked black beans, drained

6 tablespoons Maple BBQ Sauce (see recipe on page 156)

¼ cup plain nonfat Greek yogurt (optional)

Directions

1. Heat a dry large skillet over medium heat, and add the tomatoes, onions and garlic. Cook the vegetables for 5 minutes, or until they are tender and lightly browned.

2. Add the black beans and Maple BBQ Sauce, and cook over medium heat for 5 minutes, or until heated throughout.

3. Serving Suggestion: Serve topped with Greek yogurt.

Nutrition Facts (per serving without the Greek yogurt)

140 calories, 0 grams fat, 0 grams saturated fat, 0 grams trans fat, 0 milligrams cholesterol, 130 milligrams sodium, 28 grams carbohydrates, 5 grams fiber, 9 grams sugar, 7 grams protein

GUILTLESS GARLIC BREAD

Yield: 4 servings

This recipe, a healthier twist on garlic bread, is something I have been making since college!

Before:

Cheesy garlic bread tends to be loaded with butter and to go overboard on the cheese.

Skinny-Size It:

Toasted garlic bread topped with plenty of garlicky sautéed spinach and just enough light cheddar cheese has only 150 calories per slice. One slice of this Guiltless Garlic Bread also boasts 4 grams of fiber and immune-boosting vitamin A, providing 60 percent of the daily value for vitamin A.

Skinny Shopping:

When buying cheese, opt for light or reduced-fat varieties to quickly slash calories and total fat from cheesy recipes. A light option to look for is Cabot Sharp Light Cheddar Cheese, with only 70 calories and 4.5 grams total fat per ounce.

Ingredients

4 slices 100 percent whole-wheat bread

1 teaspoon extra-virgin olive oil

4 cloves garlic, peeled and minced

4 cups baby spinach

1 ounce light cheddar cheese, shredded
(such as Cabot Sharp Light Cheddar Cheese)

Directions

1. Preheat the oven to 350°F. Lightly toast the slices of bread in a toaster, then place them on a baking sheet and set aside.

2. Heat the olive oil in a large skillet over medium heat. Add the garlic and sauté until just fragrant, about 1 minute.

3. Add the spinach and sauté for 2 to 3 minutes, or until it is wilted.

4. Spread the spinach-garlic mixture on the reserved bread slices. Sprinkle the cheese on top.

5. Bake the garlic bread for 3 to 5 minutes, or until the cheese has melted. Serve warm.

Nutrition Facts (per serving)

150 calories, 4.5 grams fat, 1 gram saturated fat, 0 grams trans fat, < 5 milligrams cholesterol, 250 milligrams sodium, 22 grams carbohydrates, 4 grams fiber, 3 grams sugar, 7 grams protein

BAKED STUFFED TOMATOES

Yield: 4 servings (2 halves each)

Before:

Many recipes with the word *stuffed* in the name are loaded with calories and fat.

Skinny-Size It:

Making the stuffing for these baked tomatoes with whole-wheat panko-style bread crumbs adds crunch, and using water to soften the bread crumbs eliminates the need for added fat. Start with plain whole-wheat bread crumbs, as this allows you to add your own seasoning blend and to control the amount of added sodium in the recipe. Many seasoned bread crumbs pack over 350 milligrams of sodium per quarter cup, compared to just 23 milligrams of sodium per quarter cup of plain whole-wheat bread crumbs.

Skinny Swap:

Panko bread crumbs are Japanese-style bread crumbs. They are crunchier than regular bread crumbs and absorb less oil when fried, resulting in a lighter coating. Swap high-sodium seasoned bread crumbs for plain bread crumbs and add your own spices (but no salt) to give them pizzazz. And opt for whole-wheat varieties to add fiber to a dish!

Ingredients

1 cup unseasoned whole-wheat panko bread crumbs

1 teaspoon garlic powder

1 teaspoon dried oregano

1 teaspoon dried basil

2 tablespoons water

4 plum tomatoes

¼ cup grated Parmesan cheese

Directions

1. Preheat the oven to 350°F.
2. In a small mixing bowl, combine the bread crumbs, garlic powder, oregano and basil. Add the water and mix well.
3. Slice the tomatoes in half lengthwise and place them seeded side up in a baking dish.
4. Top each tomato half with the bread crumb mixture and sprinkle with the cheese.
5. Bake the tomatoes for 25 to 30 minutes, or until the bread crumb topping is lightly browned. Serve warm.

Nutrition Facts (per serving)

110 calories, 2 grams fat, 1 gram saturated fat, 0 grams trans fat, < 5 milligrams cholesterol, 105 milligrams sodium, 18 grams carbohydrates, 3 grams fiber, 2 grams sugar, 6 grams protein

COTTAGE VEGGIE BAKE

Yield: 8 servings

Before:

My husband and I first had this dish at a restaurant years ago, and we loved it, yet we knew it was loaded with calories and fat because of the generous amounts of bread crumbs, oil and cheese, including Parmesan and feta.

Skinny-Size It:

Back in our kitchen, I figured out how to re-create it and, as always, how to Skinny-Size It. I opted for whole-wheat panko bread crumbs, low-fat cottage cheese and crumbled blue cheese and relied on the veggies for moisture, eliminating the added oil. Each of these swaps enhanced the taste and texture of the dish, while effectively reducing the calories and the total fat. The result is a staple dish, especially in the summer, with only 110 calories and 3 grams of fat per serving.

Ingredients

Nonstick cooking spray, for greasing the baking dish

2 medium zucchini, ends cut off and sliced thin

2 medium yellow squash, ends cut off and sliced thin

4 plum tomatoes, sliced thin

1 cup low-fat cottage cheese

½ cup crumbled blue cheese

1 cup whole-wheat panko bread crumbs

Directions

1. Preheat the oven to 350°F. Lightly coat a deep 4-quart baking dish with cooking spray.

2. Place a third of the zucchini, yellow squash and tomato slices in the prepared baking dish, creating an even layer. Spoon ½ cup of the cottage cheese and ¼ cup of the blue cheese atop the veggies, and then sprinkle with ⅓ cup of the bread crumbs. Place a third of the veggie slices atop the bread crumbs, spoon the remaining ½ cup cottage cheese and ¼ cup blue cheese on top of the veggies, and sprinkle with ⅓ cup of the bread crumbs. Add a last layer of veggies and top with the remaining ⅓ cup bread crumbs.

3. Bake for 50 minutes to 1 hour, or until the vegetables are tender and the cheeses are hot. Serve at once.

Nutrition Facts (per serving)

110 calories, 3 grams fat, 2 grams saturated fat, 0 grams trans fat, 10 milligrams cholesterol, 250 milligrams sodium, 13 grams carbohydrates, 2 grams fiber, 4 grams sugar, 8 grams protein

MAPLE-GLAZED PARSNIPS

Yield: 4 servings

It is tough to Skinny size this dish since parsnips have only 55 calories and 3 grams of fiber per half cup. In this recipe the natural sweetness of parsnips is enhanced with a drizzle of pure maple syrup before baking, which also adds phenolic compounds to this vegetable and provides an antioxidant boost. Pure maple syrup has been found to possess twenty or more potential health-promoting properties. Maple syrup's concentration of antioxidants may be due in part to the fact that it is made from maple tree sap, which flows through the outer tree trunk, right under the bark, the part of the tree that soaks up the sun.

Skinny Shopping:

Parsnips, which look like white carrots and are part of the carrot family, have a light, sweet flavor. Look for them in the grocery store produce section, near the carrots.

Ingredients

1½ pounds of parsnips (about 6 medium), peeled and cut into 1-inch cubes (about 2 cups)

2 tablespoons pure maple syrup

Directions

1. Preheat the oven to 425°F.
2. Place the parsnips in a 9 x 9-inch baking dish and toss with the maple syrup to coat. Bake for 25 to 30 minutes, or until the parsnips are tender, and serve.

Nutrition Facts (per serving)

70 calories, 0 grams fat, 0 grams saturated fat, 0 grams trans fat, 0 milligrams cholesterol, 5 milligrams sodium, 17 grams carbohydrates, 3 grams fiber, 8 grams sugar, < 1 gram protein

BALSAMIC FIVE BEAN SALAD

Yield: 12 servings (¾ cup each)

Before:

Most traditional bean salads feature no more than three varieties of beans, all marinated in a sugary vinaigrette.

Skinny-Size It:

The Skinny-Size It version skimps on the amount of added sugar and relies on the lightly sweet taste of balsamic vinegar. The whole recipe of the homemade White Balsamic Vinaigrette (see recipe on page 151) in this salad has only 2 tablespoons of added sugar and each serving of this salad has only 2 grams of sugar per serving.

Skinny Tip:

Prepare this salad on the weekend, and then store it in single serving (about ¾ cup) containers for a quick side dish to grab on the go and to add to lunches throughout the week.

Ingredients

One 15½-ounce can chickpeas, drained and rinsed

One 15½-ounce can black beans, drained and rinsed

One 15½-ounce can pinto beans, drained and rinsed

One 15½-ounce can red kidney beans, drained and rinsed

1 cup frozen green beans, thawed and cooked

1 medium red bell pepper, seeded, deribbed and diced

1 small sweet onion, peeled and diced

½ cup White Balsamic Vinaigrette (see recipe on
page 151)

Directions

1. In a large mixing bowl, combine all the ingredients and
   mix well. Place the bean salad in an airtight container
   and marinate overnight.

Nutrition Facts (per serving)

160 calories, 2.5 grams fat, 0 grams saturated fat, 0 grams trans
fat, 0 milligrams cholesterol, 320 milligrams sodium, 27 grams
carbohydrates, 7 grams fiber, 2 grams sugar, 7 grams protein

SWEET POTATO FRIES

Yield: 4 servings

Before:

Sweet potatoes are low in fat and packed with vitamin A, but
once they are deep-fried, a serving can have 200 calories or
more and upwards of 11 grams of fat.

Skinny-Size It:

Roasting sliced sweet potatoes in the oven until they get
crispy is an excellent way to enjoy them, and the best part
is that they have only a fraction of the total fat and calories
found in deep-fried sweet potato fries. One serving of these
revamped sweet potato fries has 130 calories, 2.5 grams of
fat and 370 percent of the daily value for vitamin A.

Skinny Kitchen:

A spray bottle filled with extra-virgin olive oil is a perfect tool in the Skinny kitchen. A single squirt typically contains about a quarter teaspoon of oil, and spraying enables you to disperse the oil over the food or the bakeware you are preparing, so you end up using much less. Check home stores for spray bottle options.

Ingredients

4 small sweet potatoes, peeled and cut lengthwise into ¼-inch-thick fries

2 teaspoons extra-virgin olive oil

Sea salt, to taste

Directions

1. Preheat the oven to 425°F.

2. Arrange the sweet potatoes on a baking sheet in a single layer and spray or drizzle with olive oil.

3. Bake for 20 to 30 minutes, turning occasionally, or until the fries are tender in the center and crispy on the outside. Add sea salt to taste. Serve at once.

Nutrition Facts (per serving)

130 calories, 2.5 grams fat, 0 grams saturated fat, 0 grams trans fat, 0 milligrams cholesterol, 70 milligrams sodium, 26 grams carbohydrates, 4 grams fiber, 5 grams sugar, 2 grams protein

ROASTED ROSEMARY FINGERLING POTATOES

Yield: 4 servings

Before:

Potatoes are naturally fat free, but most traditional roasted potato dishes are laden with fat.

Skinny-Size It:

This recipe skimps on the amount of added oil and focuses on seasoning the potatoes with fresh rosemary, and garlic powder gives them excellent flavor, which only deepens as the potatoes roast. This recipe has just 2.5 grams of fat per serving.

Ingredients

1½ pounds unpeeled fingerling potatoes, halved lengthwise

2 teaspoons extra-virgin olive oil

1 teaspoon minced fresh rosemary

1 teaspoon garlic powder

Directions

1. Preheat the oven to 425°F.
2. On a baking sheet, sprinkle the potatoes with the olive oil, rosemary and garlic powder, and toss to coat.
3. Bake for 35 to 45 minutes, or until the potatoes are tender and their skin is lightly browned.

Nutrition Facts (per serving)

90 calories, 2.5 grams fat, 0 grams saturated fat, 0 grams trans fat, 0 milligrams cholesterol, 0 milligrams sodium, 17 grams carbohydrates, 2 grams fiber, 2 grams sugar, 3 grams protein

PINEAPPLE COLESLAW

Yield: 8 servings

Before:

Traditional homemade coleslaw and the coleslaw served in restaurants tend to be loaded with full fat mayonnaise and plenty of sugar. A single serving may have 200 calories or more, as much as 5 teaspoons of added sugar (20 grams of sugar) and 300 milligrams of sodium or more.

Skinny-Size It:

Using oil with a light flavor, such as canola oil, in place of the mayonnaise and adding pineapple for natural sweetness make for a coleslaw with less fat, a lot less sugar and only 20 milligrams of sodium per serving.

Skinny Shopping:

If you're gearing up to make coleslaw, look for bags of pre-shredded cabbage and carrots in the grocery store. They are a great time-saver!

Ingredients

¾ cup white vinegar

½ cup pineapple juice (reserved from the crushed pineapple)

¼ cup canola oil

¼ cup sugar

½ teaspoon celery seed

5 cups shredded cabbage

1 cup shredded carrots

1 cup crushed pineapple, drained (½ cup of the juice reserved)

Directions

1. Prepare the marinade by combining the vinegar, pineapple juice, canola oil, sugar and celery seed in a small saucepan. Bring to a boil over medium heat, let boil 1 minute more and then remove from the heat.

2. In a large mixing bowl, combine the cabbage, carrots and crushed pineapple. Pour the marinade over the cabbage mixture, cover and refrigerate overnight.

Nutrition Facts (per serving)

120 calories, 7 grams fat, 0.5 grams saturated fat, 0 grams trans fat, 0 milligrams cholesterol, 20 milligrams sodium, 14 grams carbohydrates, 2 grams fiber, 12 grams sugar, < 1 gram protein

CRUNCHY GARLIC BROCCOLI

Yield: 4 servings

Before:

Many broccoli dishes that are creamy or crunchy are loaded with oil, mayonnaise or cheese and thus are high in calories and fat.

Skinny-Size It:

Going easy on the oil, flavoring with garlic and using panko bread crumbs—which are lower in calories, fat and sodium compared to traditional bread crumbs—results in a crunchy, garlicky broccoli dish with only 90 calories and 3.5 grams of fat per serving.

Skinny Tip:

Garlic is an ingredient that you should always keep on hand and routinely work into your culinary routine. The phytochemical content (powerful plant compounds) of garlic has been linked to a reduced risk of certain types of cancer and to lowering cholesterol levels. A personal favorite garlic of mine is elephant garlic, which has jumbo cloves—each clove is equal to 3 or 4 regular garlic cloves—a great time-saver!

Ingredients

3 cups broccoli florets

½ cup whole-wheat panko bread crumbs

1 tablespoon garlic powder

3 cloves garlic, peeled and minced

1 tablespoon extra-virgin olive oil

Directions

1. Preheat the oven to 425°F.
2. In a medium-size mixing bowl, combine the broccoli, bread crumbs, garlic powder, minced garlic and olive oil, and toss to coat.
3. Transfer the broccoli to a baking sheet and bake for 15 minutes, or until the broccoli is cooked and the bread crumbs are crunchy.

Nutrition Facts (per serving)

90 calories, 3.5 grams fat, 0 grams saturated fat, 0 grams trans fat, 0 milligrams cholesterol, 35 milligrams sodium, 11 grams carbohydrates, 3 grams fiber, 2 grams sugar, 2 grams protein

ROASTED ASPARAGUS AND QUINOA SALAD

Yield: 6 servings

Before:

Many grain-based salads are loaded with sodium, owing largely to the dressings that flavor them.

Skinny-Size It:

The base of this salad is quinoa, a protein-packed seed that cooks up like a grain. Quinoa is a must-have for salads and side dishes. Plus, making your own vinaigrette results in only 35 milligrams of sodium and 4 grams of fat per serving—this vinaigrette enlivens salads the healthy way.

Skinny Swap:

Making your own vinaigrette is simple! This recipe combines a blend of vinegar, a small amount of extra-virgin olive oil, agave nectar (to sweeten it up) and plenty of fresh parsley and garlic. Try this Skinny-Size It vinaigrette on other salads, too.

Ingredients

16 spears asparagus, trimmed

1 cup quinoa

2 cups water

¼ cup balsamic vinegar

2 tablespoons red wine vinegar

1 tablespoon extra-virgin olive oil

1 tablespoon agave nectar

¼ cup minced fresh parsley

1 teaspoon minced garlic

3 Roma tomatoes, diced

5 pitted black olives, sliced

Fresh parsley sprigs, for garnish

Directions

1. Preheat the oven to 350°F.

2. Place the asparagus on a baking sheet and roast in the oven for 10 to 15 minutes, or until they are tender and lightly browned. Remove the asparagus to a large plate and let cool. Then cut the asparagus diagonally into 1-inch pieces and set aside.

3. While the asparagus are cooling, rinse the quinoa in a fine-mesh strainer to wash away the saponins, a naturally occurring soap-like substance that is on the outside of the quinoa and has a bitter flavor.

4. Combine the quinoa and the water in a medium saucepan and bring to a boil over medium heat. Reduce the heat and simmer the quinoa for 15 minutes, or until the water is absorbed. When the quinoa is done, the outer translucent germ layer will separate from the seed.

5. In a small mixing bowl, combine the balsamic vinegar, red wine vinegar, olive oil and agave nectar and mix well with a whisk. Add the parsley and garlic, and then stir in the cooked quinoa.

6. Transfer the quinoa to a serving plate and top with the reserved asparagus, the tomatoes and the black olives. Garnish with the parsley sprigs, and serve.

Nutrition Facts (per serving)

150 calories, 4 grams fat, 0 grams saturated fat, 0 grams trans fat, 0 milligrams cholesterol, 35 milligrams sodium, 24 grams carbohydrates, 3 grams fiber, 7 grams sugar, 5 grams protein

CALABACITAS

Yield: 6 servings

The Spanish word *calabacitas* means "zucchini." A traditional Southwestern dish that utilizes zucchini and yellow squash as the base bears the same name. Calabacitas is an excellent side dish and taco filling.

Before:

Most Calabacitas recipes start with a hefty quantity of oil or butter and end with half-and-half and cheese, which moves otherwise healthy summer squash into the heavyweight category.

Skinny-Size It:

Keeping the main emphasis of the recipe on zucchini and yellow squash, leaving behind the half-and-half and cheese, and adding beans put this dish in the Skinny-Size It category, with only 120 calories and 8 grams of fiber per serving.

Ingredients

1 large sweet onion, peeled and diced

3 cloves garlic, peeled and minced

2 cups diced yellow squash

2 cups diced zucchini

2 cups fresh corn (frozen corn works great
if fresh is not available)

One 15-ounce can black beans, rinsed and drained

1 medium red bell pepper, seeded, deribbed
and diced

1 medium green bell pepper, seeded, deribbed
and diced

½ jalapeño pepper, seeded and diced (optional)

½ teaspoon freshly ground black pepper

½ teaspoon sea salt

Directions

1. In a large Dutch oven or soup pot, combine the
   onions and garlic, and sauté over medium heat until
   the onions are tender, about 5 to 7 minutes.
2. Add the yellow squash, zucchini, corn, black beans,
   and red and green bell peppers and stir. Add the
   jalapeño, if desired, and season with pepper and
   sea salt.
3. Cover and cook the vegetables until they are tender,
   about 10 minutes.

Nutrition Facts (per serving)

120 calories, 0.5 grams fat, 0 grams saturated fat, 0 grams trans
fat, 0 milligrams cholesterol, 200 milligrams sodium, 23 grams
carbohydrates, 8 grams fiber, 3 grams sugar, 7 grams protein

TABBOULEH

Yield: 6 servings

Before:

Tabbouleh is a traditional Middle Eastern dish that is typically made with bulgur wheat or couscous. The only caution is that many recipes have a large quantity of olive oil in them, which kicks up the calories and fat.

Skinny-Size It:

Make tabbouleh the Skinny-Size It way and keep the traditional ingredients, including cucumber, tomato, parsley and mint, while cutting the olive oil back to only 1 tablespoon. Skimping on the oil and relying on the fresh flavors of the vegetables, lemon juice and vinegar keep the calories at only 90 per serving, which is less than half found in the typical serving of tabbouleh.

Ingredients

½ cup uncooked bulgur wheat, cooked per package instructions

1 medium cucumber, seeded and diced

1 pint cherry tomatoes, stems removed and halved

¼ cup minced fresh parsley

¼ cup minced fresh mint

2 tablespoons white vinegar

1 tablespoon freshly squeezed lemon juice

1 tablespoon extra-virgin olive oil

1 teaspoon garlic powder

Directions

1. In a medium mixing bowl, combine the cooked bulgur wheat, cucumbers, tomatoes, parsley and mint.

2. In a small mixing bowl, whisk together the vinegar, lemon juice, olive oil and garlic powder. Add the vinegar mixture to the bulgur wheat and vegetables, and stir well.

3. Chill the tabbouleh for 2 to 4 hours (or overnight), and then serve.

Nutrition Facts (per serving)

90 calories, 2.5 grams fat, 0 grams saturated fat, 0 grams trans fat, 0 milligrams cholesterol, 5 milligrams sodium, 16 grams carbohydrates, 3 grams fiber, 2 grams sugar, 3 grams protein

5

....

Snacks
and Appetizers

S kinny Rule #79 for parties and travel is "Lighten Up Party Heavyweights!" The snack and appetizer recipes in this chapter do just that. Who wants to go to a party and just nibble on plain old celery sticks? There are plenty of healthy ways to enjoy traditionally wicked appetizers and filling snacks, such as guiltless Chicken Wing Dip, which goes great with celery sticks and other sliced vegetables! These Skinny-Size It snacks and appetizers won't leave you or your guests feeling deprived.

Some of the side dish recipes in this book, such as Guiltless Garlic Bread, Baked Stuffed Tomatoes, Sweet Potato Fries and Crunchy Garlic Broccoli, can double as snacks or appetizers. From the Sauces, Dressings and Dips chapter, Salsa-Mole,

Ranch Dressing, Skinny-Size It Hummus and Yogurt Tzatziki are perfect to pair with sliced vegetables, baked whole-grain corn chips and whole-wheat pita wedges for a healthy snack. And the drinks and smoothies in Chapter 7 are great accompaniments to your snack and appetizer lineup.

POTATO SKINNIES

Yield: 8 servings (2 potato skins each)

Before:

A half order of some restaurant loaded potato skins can have upwards of 80 grams of fat. Even if you are splitting the potato skins among a few people, you would still be looking at over 20 grams of fat before your main dish even arrives.

Skinny-Size It:

Making your own potato skins is often a much healthier option. Plus potato skins are loaded with minerals—one serving of Potato Skinnies has 23 percent of the daily value for copper, 24 percent for iron and 18 percent for manganese. Topping potato skins with light cheese adds lots of cheesy flavor but only half the fat and saturated fat. Serving the skins with plain nonfat Greek yogurt and fresh salsa is a perfect way to dress them without piling on any fat.

Ingredients

8 medium russet potatoes

2 ounces light cheddar cheese, shredded
(such as Cabot Sharp Light Cheddar Cheese)

¼ cup minced scallions

2 slices cooked bacon, crumbled

¼ cup plain nonfat Greek yogurt

¼ cup fresh tomato salsa of your choice

Directions

1. Preheat the oven to 350°F. Prepare the potato skins by piercing the potatoes and placing them on a baking sheet. Bake the potatoes for 1 hour, or until they are tender. Remove the potatoes to a large platter and let cool.

2. Once the potatoes are cool, slice them in half lengthwise and remove most of the potato flesh (which can be refrigerated and reserved for another use).

3. Arrange the potato skins on the baking sheet skin side down. Top the skins with the cheese, scallions and bacon.

4. Bake the potato skins for 7 to 10 minutes, or until they are hot and the cheese is melted.

5. In a small bowl, mix together the Greek yogurt and salsa. Serve it as a dip with the potato skins.

Nutrition Facts (per serving)

150 calories, 2 grams fat, 1 gram saturated fat, 0 grams trans fat, 5 milligrams cholesterol, 125 milligrams sodium, 28 grams carbohydrates, 5 grams fiber, 1 gram sugar, 6 grams protein

BAKED APPLE PIE PARFAITS

Yield: 2 servings

Before:

Apple pies and apple crisps can be loaded with sugar and fat.

Skinny-Size It:

Taking a twist on the traditional and making a baked apple dish that is lightly sweetened and contains plenty of cinnamon adds a ton of flavor without all the added sugar and calories.

Ingredients

2 medium McIntosh, Golden Delicious (or other varieties good for baking) apples , peeled, cored and sliced

1 tablespoon agave nectar

1 teaspoon ground cinnamon

6 ounces low-fat vanilla yogurt

¼ cup KIND Healthy Grains Maple Walnut Clusters with Chia & Quinoa or similar granola with 130 calories and 3.5 grams fat or less per serving

Directions

1. Preheat the oven to 350°F.
2. Place the apple slices in a small mixing bowl, add the agave nectar and cinnamon, and toss to coat. Transfer the apples to a baking sheet.
3. Bake the apples for 20 to 25 minutes, or until they are tender.
4. Serve the baked apples over vanilla yogurt and garnish with the granola.

Nutrition Facts (per serving)

230 calories, 1.5 grams fat, 0 grams saturated fat, 0 grams trans fat, 0 milligrams cholesterol, 65 milligrams sodium, 53 grams carbohydrates, 7 grams fiber, 39 grams sugar, 5 grams protein

APPLE CINNAMON CHIA SWIRL PUDDING

Yield: 4 servings

Before:

A serving of pudding prepared with whole milk is full of fat and calories, with most of those calories coming from sugar.

Skinny-Size It:

Making pudding with chia seeds upgrades the quality of the calories. This pudding is an excellent snack or dessert. Each serving has 12 grams of fat and delivers heart-helping omega-3 fats and 14 grams of fiber.

Skinny Shopping:

Look for chia seeds in the baking aisle or health food section of your grocery store.

Ingredients

2 cups vanilla almond milk

½ cup chia seeds

1 tablespoon pure maple syrup

1 teaspoon ground cinnamon, plus 1 teaspoon
for sprinkling

2 medium McIntosh, Golden Delicious (or other
varieties good for baking) apples, peeled,
cored and diced

¼ cup plain nonfat Greek yogurt

Directions

1. In a quart-size container, such as a canning jar,
combine the almond milk, chia seeds, maple syrup
and 1 teaspoon of the cinnamon. Stir well, cover and
refrigerate overnight (or for 8 to 10 hours) to allow
the mixture to thicken to pudding consistency.

2. Spoon the pudding into 4 serving bowls and top with
the apples and Greek yogurt. Sprinkle the remaining
1 teaspoon cinnamon on top, and serve at once.

Nutrition Facts (per serving)

220 calories, 12 grams fat, 1 gram saturated fat, 0 grams trans
fat, 0 milligrams cholesterol, 100 milligrams sodium, 30 grams
carbohydrates, 14 grams fiber, 15 grams sugar, 6 grams protein

CHICKEN WING DIP

Yield: 8 servings

Before:

Just the words *chicken wing* should send up a caution flag. Many
chicken wing dip recipes are loaded with fat and calories.

Skinny-Size It:

Using homemade Ranch Dressing (see recipe on page 147), which is super simple to make, and light versions of cream cheese and cheddar cheese moves this dip recipe out of the red zone and into the healthier zone. The savings per serving with the Skinny swaps are 60 calories, 11 grams of fat and 445 milligrams of sodium compared to the traditional recipe.

Skinny Shopping:

Look for Cabot Sharp Light Cheddar Cheese in the dairy case, as it has half the fat compared to regular cheddar cheese, melts well and tastes marvelous. You won't even miss the fat!

Ingredients

8 ounces light cream cheese (1 brick)

One 12 ½-ounce can white chicken

½ cup Ranch Dressing (see recipe on page 147)

¼ cup hot sauce

½ cup light cheddar cheese, shredded (2 ounces)

Directions

1. Preheat the oven to 350°F.
2. Melt the cream cheese in a medium saucepan over medium heat. Stir in the chicken, Ranch Dressing and hot sauce.

3. Transfer the chicken–cream cheese mixture to an 8 x 8-inch baking dish and top with the shredded cheese.
4. Bake for 15 minutes, or until the cheese is bubbly.
5. Serving Suggestion: Serve the dip with sliced carrots, celery sticks and multigrain tortilla chips.

Nutrition Facts (per serving without the carrots, celery and multigrain tortilla chips)

150 calories, 10 grams fat, 4.5 grams saturated fat, 0 grams trans fat, 45 milligrams cholesterol, 510 milligrams sodium, 4 grams carbohydrates, 0 grams fiber, 2 grams sugar, 10 grams protein

CHEWY APRICOT GRANOLA

Yield: 12 servings

Before:

Granola is one of those foods that seems like it should always be healthy, yet often it is loaded with fat, sugar and calories and is almost like eating a cookie.

Skinny Tip:

This granola and the PB Pretzel Granola (see recipe on page 136) are so delicious! After the granola cools, divide it into single serving bags or containers to keep portion sizes in check! It makes a great snack or topping for low-fat yogurt.

Skinny-Size It:

Making your own granola is simple and allows you the flexibility of adjusting the amount and type of added fat and sugar while loading it up with plenty of fruit. Chewy Apricot Granola has 4 grams of fiber, 8 grams of fat and 210 calories per serving, with a majority of the sugar coming from dried apricots.

Ingredients

Parchment paper, for lining the baking dish

1 cup old-fashioned oats, plus 1 cup left whole

2 cups diced dried apricots

¼ cup sunflower seed kernels

⅓ cup honey

3 tablespoons unsalted margarine, melted

2 tablespoons coconut oil, melted

Directions

1. Preheat the oven to 350°F. Prepare a 9 x 9-inch baking dish by lining it with parchment paper.

2. Place 1 cup of the oats in a food processor and pulse until they resemble flour.

3. In a large mixing bowl, combine the oat "flour," the remaining 1 cup whole oats, apricots, sunflower seeds, honey, margarine and coconut oil, and mix well.

4. Transfer the oat mixture to the prepared baking dish and spread it out evenly.

5. Bake for 20 minutes, or until the granola is lightly browned. Cool the granola and store it in an airtight container, or divide it into single servings and store in airtight containers.

Nutrition Facts (per serving)

210 calories, 8 grams fat, 3 grams saturated fat, 0 grams trans fat, 0 milligrams cholesterol, 25 milligrams sodium, 35 grams carbohydrates, 4 grams fiber, 23 grams sugar, 3 grams protein

PB PRETZEL GRANOLA

Yield: 12 servings

Before:

This recipe was inspired by a peanut butter pretzel bar that I love. I wanted to develop a higher fiber and lower sugar version.

Skinny-Size It:

An old-fashioned oats–based granola with natural peanut butter and agave nectar provides double the fiber compared to the bar I love. Plus, there is 1 teaspoon less sugar than the bar, and every teaspoon of sugar saved is a good thing.

Ingredients

Parchment paper, for lining the baking dish

2 ½ cups whole-wheat pretzels (such as Snyder's of Hanover), chopped

1 cup old-fashioned oats, plus 1 cup left whole

2 tablespoons chia seeds

⅓ cup creamy natural peanut butter

⅓ cup extra-virgin olive oil

⅓ cup agave nectar

Directions

1. Preheat the oven to 350°F. Prepare a 9 x 9-inch baking dish by lining it with parchment paper.

2. Place the pretzels in a food processor and process until they are coarsely ground. Remove the ground pretzels to a large mixing bowl. Place 1 cup of the oats in the food processor and pulse until they resemble flour. Add the oat "flour" to the pretzels in the mixing bowl. Then stir in the remaining 1 cup whole oats and the chia seeds, mix well and set aside.

3. In a small saucepan, combine the peanut butter, olive oil and agave nectar. Heat the mixture over medium heat, stirring frequently, until warmed through and well combined.

4. Stir the peanut butter mixture into the reserved oat-pretzel mixture and mix well.

5. Transfer the peanut butter–oat mixture to the prepared baking dish and spread it out evenly.

6. Bake for 20 minutes, or until the granola is lightly browned. Cool the granola and store it in an airtight container, or divide it into single servings and store in airtight containers.

Nutrition Facts (per serving)

210 calories, 12 grams fat, 1.5 grams saturated fat, 0 grams trans fat, 0 milligrams cholesterol, 45 milligrams sodium, 23 grams carbohydrates, 4 grams fiber, 5 grams sugar, 5 grams protein

SOUTHWESTERN PIZZA

Yield: 14 servings (1 slice each)

Before:

Pizza is often removed from meal plans because of its high calorie and fat content. Yet with the right Skinny swaps, you can easily keep pizza in your repertoire.

Skinny-Size It:

Start with whole-wheat pizza dough for added fiber and a flavorful crust. Then top the dough with a bean-based salsa for additional belly-filling fiber and excellent flavor, and adorn it with healthy toppings, like fresh vegetables, beans and part-skim mozzarella.

Skinny Tip:

When selecting cheese, opt for part-skim or 50 percent reduced-fat varieties, which cuts down on the saturated fat. Or make it vegan by swapping dairy mozzarella cheese for Daiya Mozzarella Style Shreds.

Ingredients

Nonstick cooking spray, for greasing the baking sheet
(omit if using a pizza stone)

1 whole-wheat pizza dough ball
(homemade or store-bought)

1 cup black bean and corn salsa

1¼ cups part-skim mozzarella cheese, shredded

1½ cups cooked black beans

1 small orange bell pepper, seeded, deribbed and
thinly sliced

2 medium scallions, root ends trimmed and thinly sliced

Skinny Kitchen:

If you don't already have a pizza stone, you
might consider getting one. A pizza stone is a
great addition to a Skinny kitchen. It bakes up
pizza crust perfectly.

Directions

1. Preheat the oven to 450°F. Coat a baking sheet
   with cooking spray or preheat a pizza stone for
   15 minutes.
2. Roll out the dough on a clean, lightly floured work
   surface to the desired shape. Place the dough on
   the baking sheet or prepared pizza stone.
3. Top the dough with the salsa and then the mozzarella.
   Then top the cheese with the beans, peppers and
   scallions, distributing them evenly.
4. Bake the pizza for 8 to 10 minutes, or until the cheese
   is melted. Cut into 14 slices, and serve at once.

Nutrition Facts (per serving)

210 calories, 5 grams fat, 2.5 grams saturated fat, 0 grams trans
fat, 10 milligrams cholesterol, 450 milligrams sodium, 33 grams
carbohydrates, 4 grams fiber, 4 grams sugar, 11 grams protein

POT STICKERS

Yield: 10 servings

Before:

Pot stickers are typically filled with meat and veggies and then fried in oil.

Skinny-Size It:

A 100 percent vegetable-based filling, which is stuffed into egg roll wrappers, keeps this appetizer at only 110 calories per pot sticker. The garlic and ginger impart a vibrant flavor to the vegetable filling, so much so that it can double as a delicious side dish to serve with an Asian-style meal.

Ingredients

1 pound bok choy, end removed and sliced thin
(about 4 cups)

1 medium carrot, peeled and cut into 1-inch julienne strips

4 cloves garlic, peeled and minced

2 tablespoons lite soy sauce

½ teaspoon minced fresh ginger

10 egg roll wrappers

Nonstick cooking spray, for greasing the skillet

¼ cup Honey-Sesame Soy Sauce (see recipe on
page 152)

Directions

1. Heat a large skillet over medium heat and add the bok choy, carrots, garlic, soy sauce and ginger. Sweat the vegetables for 2 to 3 minutes, or until the bok choy is wilted.

2. Arrange the egg roll wrappers on a clean work surface. Pour a little water in a small bowl and place it near the work surface. Lay a wrapper flat on the work surface. Place 2 tablespoons of the vegetable mixture in the center of the wrapper. Fold the bottom of the wrapper over the filling and then fold in the sides. Moisten the top edge of the wrapper and then roll the wrapper up tightly, pressing to seal the moistened edge. Repeat until all the wrappers have been filled and rolled.

3. Coat a medium skillet with cooking spray and heat over medium heat. Working in batches, cook the pot stickers, rotating them in the skillet, until they are golden brown, about 2 minutes each side. (Coat the skillet with cooking spray in between batches.)

4. Serve the pot stickers at once with the Honey-Sesame Soy Sauce as a dip.

Nutrition Facts (per serving)

110 calories, 0.5 grams fat, 0 grams saturated fat, 0 grams trans fat, < 5 milligrams cholesterol, 390 milligrams sodium, 21 grams carbohydrates, 2 grams fiber, 6 grams sugar, 4 grams protein

FALAFEL

Yield: 6 servings

Before:

Falafel is a mixture of ground chickpeas and spices that is formed into small balls or patties and typically fried in vegetable oil, which kicks up the calories of this otherwise low-fat dish.

Skinny-Size It:
Panfrying falafel with cooking spray will crisp it up without adding tons of fat and calories. Each serving has 160 calories, 2 grams of fat and 6 grams of fiber.

Skinny Tip:

Falafel tastes great on whole-wheat pita, topped with fresh vegetables, such as romaine lettuce, tomatoes and cucumbers, and served with tzatziki.

Ingredients

One 15 ½-ounce can chickpeas, rinsed and drained

1 cup diced sweet onion

2 tablespoons minced fresh parsley

2 tablespoons minced fresh cilantro

4 cloves garlic, peeled and coarsely chopped

1 teaspoon ground cumin

4 tablespoons whole-wheat flour

Nonstick cooking spray, for greasing the skillet

½ cup Yogurt Tzatziki (see recipe on page 167)

Directions

1. In a food processor, combine the chickpeas, onions, parsley, cilantro, garlic and cumin. Pulse until the chickpeas are broken up but not pureed.
2. Add the flour gradually and continue to pulse until the chickpea mixture starts to stick together.

Once the mixture can be formed into a small patty, transfer it to a medium-size mixing bowl, cover and refrigerate for 2 to 4 hours (or overnight).

3. Using your hands, form the falafel mixture into 1-inch patties.

4. Lightly coat a large skillet with cooking spray and heat over medium heat. Working in batches, cook the falafel patties for 3 to 5 minutes per side, or until they are light golden brown. (Lightly coat the skillet with cooking spray in between batches, if needed.)

5. Serve the falafel at once with the Yogurt Tzatziki as a dip.

Nutrition Facts (per serving)

160 calories, 2 grams fat, 0 grams saturated fat, 0 grams trans fat, 0 milligrams cholesterol, 115 milligrams sodium, 29 grams carbohydrates, 6 grams fiber, 5 grams sugar, 9 grams protein

PINEAPPLE HONEY SPICE CASHEWS

Yield: 10 servings

Before:

Many store-bought glazed nuts start out as roasted nuts that have added oil and salt. Then they are sweetened with sugar alone.

Skinny-Size It:

Starting out with raw cashews rather than roasted keeps the sodium to about half that of the store-bought varieties of glazed nuts, and adding dried fruit and honey in place of some of the sugar brings in more complex flavors.

Ingredients

Parchment paper, for lining the baking sheet

1½ cups raw cashews

½ cup diced dried pineapple

1 tablespoon honey

1 tablespoon sugar

1 tablespoon water

½ teaspoon chipotle chili powder

¼ teaspoon ground cumin

¼ teaspoon sea salt

Directions

1. Line a baking sheet with parchment paper.
2. Place the cashews in a medium skillet and cook, stirring frequently, over medium heat for 3 to 5 minutes, or until lightly toasted.
3. Combine the remaining ingredients in a small microwave-safe bowl and microwave on high for 30 seconds. Add the pineapple-honey mixture to the cashews in the skillet and cook over medium heat for 2 minutes, stirring constantly.
4. Transfer the glazed cashews to the prepared baking sheet, spread them out in a single layer and let stand for 10 minutes. Serve the Pineapple Honey Spice Cashews or store in an airtight container.

Nutrition Facts (per serving)

130 calories, 9 grams fat, 0.5 grams saturated fat, 0 grams trans fat, 0 milligrams cholesterol, 80 milligrams sodium, 10 grams carbohydrates, 2 grams fiber, 7 grams sugar, 4 grams protein

6

....

Sauces, Dressings and Dips

The majority of sauces, dressings and dips are packed with calories, fat and sodium. While making your own may seem like a daunting task, most sauces, dressings and dips come together in a matter of minutes, and once you have stocked up on Skinny essentials (see Stocking Your Skinny Kitchen on page xii), their preparation will become even easier. The best part about making your own sauces, dressings and dips is that you can select the quantity and the quality of the oil and add plenty of flavor with fresh herbs and spices while skipping tons of added salt.

SALSA-MOLE

Yield: 12 servings (⅓ cup each)

Before:

Avocados are full of healthy, belly-slimming unsaturated fat, yet they pack a lot of calories and fat. In fact, each avocado has about 26 grams of fat, and 17 grams of that fat is mono-unsaturated (belly-slimming) fat. When it comes to snacking on guacamole or adding it to tacos, you can pile on the calories in a hurry.

Skinny-Size It:

Mashing avocados with salsa and diced fresh tomatoes and onions is a perfect way to enjoy guacamole, while cutting down on the calories per serving. Salsa-Mole is quick and easy, and I have my sister to thank for this inspiring recipe!

Skinny Tip:

To ascertain if an avocado is ripe, press the skin lightly with your thumb. The avocado should be firm, with a slight give. If the avocado is mushy or soft in spots, this indicates that it is overripe.

Ingredients

2 medium ripe Hass avocados, halved, pits removed and peeled

1 cup fresh salsa of your choice

½ cup diced tomato

½ cup diced sweet onion

Directions

1. Place the avocado halves in a medium mixing bowl, and mash them with a fork, leaving small chunks.

2. Stir in the salsa, and then fold in the tomatoes and onions. Serve at once as a dip with carrot slices or multigrain tortilla chips or as a topping for Crunchy Tacos (see recipe on page 72).

Nutrition Facts (per serving)

70 calories, 5 grams fat, 1 gram saturated fat, 0 grams trans fat, 0 milligrams cholesterol, 130 milligrams sodium, 6 grams carbohydrates, 3 grams fiber, 2 grams sugar, 1 gram protein

RANCH DRESSING

Yield: 1 cup (16 tablespoons)

Before:

Ranch dressing is one dressing that you would not expect to find in a Skinny-Size It book, given its reputation for being high in calories, fat and sodium. However, with the right Skinny swaps, ranch dressing can be a great option for dipping veggies and using in dishes and on salads.

Skinny-Size It:

Use a mixture of reduced-fat mayonnaise, low-fat milk and light sour cream to make the perfect base for this dressing, and then add fresh flavors with dill, parsley and garlic powder.

Ingredients

¼ cup low-fat milk plus 1 tablespoon white vinegar (buttermilk)

¼ cup reduced-fat mayonnaise

¼ cup light sour cream

1 tablespoon minced fresh dill

1 tablespoon minced fresh parsley

1 teaspoon garlic powder

Directions

1. In a salad dressing shaker or a small mixing bowl, combine all the ingredients, and shake or whisk, mixing thoroughly.

2. Serve the dressing or store it in an airtight container in the refrigerator for up to 7 days.

Nutrition Facts (per serving)

15 calories, 0.5 grams fat, 0 grams saturated fat, 0 grams trans fat, 0 milligrams cholesterol, 30 milligrams sodium, 1 gram carbohydrates, 0 grams fiber, 0 grams sugar, 0 grams protein

SKINNY-SIZE IT HUMMUS

Yield: 8 servings (¼ cup each)

Before:

Store-bought hummus generally has about double the amount of sodium (150 milligrams in just 2 tablespoons) found in homemade hummus made with no added salt.

Skinny-Size It:

Keeping the right ingredients on hand makes it simple to whip up a batch of hummus. Skinny-Size It Hummus has just 150 milligrams of sodium in a serving (¼ cup, or 4 tablespoons). You can substitute cooked dried chickpeas for the canned chickpeas in this recipe to further cut down on the sodium. One of the key ingredients in hummus is tahini (sesame seed paste), which adds a nuttiness and helps give it a smooth consistency. Note: Add ¼ cup black olives or roasted red peppers to the blender along with the other hummus ingredients to switch up the flavor.

Ingredients

One 15½-ounce can chickpeas, rinsed and drained

1 tablespoon tahini

1 tablespoon freshly squeezed lemon juice

1 clove garlic, peeled

½ teaspoon ground cumin

Directions

1. In a blender or food processor, combine all the ingredients and process until smooth.
2. Serve the hummus or store it in an airtight container in the refrigerator for up to 7 days.

Nutrition Facts (per serving)

70 calories, 1.5 grams fat, 0 grams saturated fat, 0 grams trans fat, 0 milligrams cholesterol, 150 milligrams sodium, 12 grams carbohydrates, 2 grams fiber, 0 grams sugar, 3 grams protein

APPLESAUCE

Yield: 8 servings (½ cup each)

Before:

Many applesauce recipes have ½ cup of added sugar, which is equal to 24 teaspoons' worth of added sugar.

Skinny-Size It:

Let applesauce get its sweetness from the apples alone and you will do away with 8 to 9 grams of added sugar per serving, which is 2 teaspoons' worth of sugar. If you find your applesauce is too tart, which depends on the variety of apples used, sprinkle ½ teaspoon of cinnamon and ¼ teaspoon of sugar on top of each serving for a hint of extra sweetness.

Skinny Shopping:

Choose a mix of sweeter apple varieties to maximize flavor. The following apples are known for their sweetness: Cameo, Cortland, Empire, Macoun and McIntosh.

Ingredients

9 medium apples, peeled, cored and cut into quarters
(see varieties under Skinny Shopping)

½ cup water

Directions

1. Place the apples in a large pot and add the water. Bring the apples to a boil over medium heat. Reduce the heat, cover and allow the apples to simmer for 10 minutes, or until they are tender enough to be mashed.

2. Transfer the apples and their juices to a large mixing bowl and mash them with a fork or a potato masher. Cover the bowl and chill the applesauce in the refrigerator for up to 7 days.

Nutrition Facts (per serving)

70 calories, 0 grams fat, 0 grams saturated fat, 0 grams trans fat, 0 milligrams cholesterol, 0 milligrams sodium, 18 grams carbohydrates, 2 grams fiber, 15 grams sugar, 0 grams protein

WHITE BALSAMIC VINAIGRETTE

Yield: ½ cup (8 tablespoons)

Before:

When it comes to store-bought dressings that are oil based, it is difficult to know the quantity and the quality of the oil in the bottle.

Skinny-Size It:

Make your own vinaigrette and control the quality of the oil by using extra-virgin olive oil, the oil that comes from the first press of the olives, making it the most nutrient rich and flavorful of all the olive oils. A key to making your own healthy salad dressing is adjusting the ratio of oil to vinegar: use twice as much vinegar as oil. Most dressings contain the opposite—twice as much oil as vinegar.

Ingredients

¼ cup white balsamic vinegar

2 tablespoons extra-virgin olive oil

2 tablespoons sugar or agave nectar

½ teaspoon garlic powder

Freshly cracked black pepper, to taste

151

Directions

1. In a small mixing bowl, combine all the ingredients and whisk, mixing thoroughly.
2. Serve the vinaigrette or store it in an airtight container in the refrigerator for up to 7 days.

Nutrition Facts (per serving)

45 calories, 3.5 grams fat, 0 grams saturated fat, 0 grams trans fat, 0 milligrams cholesterol, 0 milligrams sodium, 4 grams carbohydrates, 0 grams fiber, 2 grams sugar, 0 grams protein

HONEY-SESAME SOY SAUCE

Yield: 1 cup (16 tablespoons)

Before:

Many prepared Asian-style sauces with a soy base are loaded with sodium.

Skinny-Size It:

Make your own with lite soy sauce and lower the sodium content substantially.

Skinny Tip:

Store homemade soy-based sauces in airtight containers in the refrigerator!

Ingredients

¹/₂ cup lite soy sauce

2 tablespoons honey

2 tablespoons rice vinegar

2 tablespoons sesame oil

2 tablespoons water

Directions

1. In a small mixing bowl, combine all the ingredients and whisk, mixing well.

2. Serve the soy sauce or store it in an airtight container in the refrigerator for up to 7 days.

Nutrition Facts (per serving)

30 calories, 1.5 grams total fat, 0 grams saturated fat, 0 grams trans fat, 0 milligrams cholesterol, 280 milligrams sodium, 3 grams carbohydrates, 0 grams fiber, 3 grams sugar, 1 gram protein

WHIPPED PINEAPPLE DIP

Yield: 1 cup (16 tablespoons)

Before:

This recipe was actually created as a Skinny frosting for the Carrot Cake Muffins, but it wound up being the perfect fruit dip. Fruit dips can be high in fat and a sneaky source of added sugar!

Skinny-Size It:

Stick with light whipped cream cheese as the foundation for your dip and add only crushed pineapple for sweetness. The result is a Skinny dip that is great with fresh fruit or even as a spread on whole-wheat crackers and has only 30 calories per serving.

Ingredients

8 ounces light cream cheese, softened

½ cup crushed pineapple (with juice)

Directions

1. Place the cream cheese in a small mixing bowl and whip with a hand mixer or by hand until smooth, about 1 minute.
2. Stir in the pineapple.
3. Serve this dip with sliced fresh fruit or whole-wheat crackers.

Nutrition Facts (per serving)

30 calories, 2 grams total fat, 1.5 grams saturated fat, 0 grams trans fat, 5 milligrams cholesterol, 65 milligrams sodium, 2 grams carbohydrates, 0 grams fiber, 2 grams sugar, 1 gram protein

BANANA MAPLE SYRUP

Yield: 12 servings (2 tablespoons each)

Before:

All the calories in maple syrup come from sugar. It is easy to pour the maple syrup on pancakes or other breakfast foods without realizing that each 1–fluid ounce (2 tablespoons) serving has 74 calories, 19 grams of carbs and 17 grams of sugar.

Skinny-Size It:

Stretch your syrup and lower its sugar content and calories by blending in fresh fruit. This syrup, which features fresh bananas, goes great with Very Banana Pancakes (see recipe on page 23). The result is a syrup with half the sugar of pure maple syrup and only 40 calories per serving.

Ingredients

2 small bananas

⅓ cup pure maple syrup

Directions

1. In a food processor or blender, combine the bananas and maple syrup, and blend until smooth.

Nutrition Facts (per serving)

40 calories, 0 grams total fat, 0 grams saturated fat, 0 grams trans fat, 0 milligrams cholesterol, 0 milligrams sodium, 10 grams carbohydrates, 0 grams fiber, 7 grams sugar, 0 grams protein

BLUEBERRY MAPLE SYRUP

Yield: 12 servings (2 tablespoons each)

Before:

Plain and simple, pure maple syrup is pure sugar.

Skinny-Size It:

Transforming pure maple syrup into fruit syrup using fresh fruit is so quick and simple to do! This blueberry syrup goes perfectly with Blueberry Buckwheat Pancakes (see recipe on page 21).

Skinny Tip:

Try your own fruit and syrup combinations to develop your own Skinny-Size It syrup.

Ingredients

1 cup fresh or frozen blueberries

⅓ cup pure maple syrup

Directions

1. In a food processor or blender, combine the blueberries and maple syrup, and blend until smooth.

Nutrition Facts (per serving)

35 calories, 0 grams total fat, 0 grams saturated fat, 0 grams trans fat, 0 milligrams cholesterol, 0 milligrams sodium, 8 grams carbohydrates, 0 grams fiber, 7 grams sugar, 0 grams protein

MAPLE BBQ SAUCE

Yield: 28 servings (1 tablespoon each)

Before:

Rule #3 in *The Skinny Rules* says, "Skip the Sauce," because store-bought sauces are often loaded with sodium and sugar. Store-bought barbecue sauces generally have about 300 to 400 milligrams of sodium per serving and 10 to 12 grams of sugar, which tends to be processed high fructose corn syrup.

Skinny-Size It:

This recipe is my husband's and the most delicious BBQ sauce! It gains its sweetness from pure maple syrup—which research has found to have antioxidant benefits—and flavor from garlic powder, pepper, dry mustard and lemon juice. Ketchup, an ingredient in this barbecue sauce, already has plenty of salt in it, so there is no need to add more salt to this recipe. If you rein in the table salt, then you wind up with a barbecue sauce that has about one-third of the sodium compared to your average store-bought version. In this Skinny barbecue sauce, while sugar is sugar, at least the sugar added is pure maple syrup with some antioxidant benefits.

Skinny Tip:

A word of caution: Even though you can control the added salt and sugar when you make your own barbecue sauce, it's not a green light to go crazy with the portions, so keep your serving size to the equivalent of a small shot glass, which equals about 1 tablespoon.

Ingredients

1 cup ketchup

½ cup pure maple syrup

2 tablespoons freshly squeezed lemon juice

1 teaspoon dry mustard

1 teaspoon freshly ground black pepper

1 teaspoon garlic powder

1 teaspoon liquid smoke

Directions

1. Combine all the ingredients in a small saucepan and cook over medium heat, stirring frequently, until the sauce is about to boil. Lower the heat to low and simmer, stirring frequently, for 20 minutes.

Nutrition Facts (per serving)

30 calories, 0 grams total fat, 0 grams saturated fat, 0 grams trans fat, 0 milligrams cholesterol, 130 milligrams sodium, 6 grams carbohydrates, 0 grams fiber, 5 grams sugar, 0 grams protein

SPIEDIE MARINADE

Yield: 1 cup (16 tablespoons)

Before:

Marinades follow the same rules as salad dressings, and therefore, making them yourself allows you to control the quality of the oil and the amount of sodium.

Skinny-Size It:

This marinade contains extra-virgin olive oil and is flavored with plenty of spices and just a small amount of sea salt. The sodium content of this Spiedie Marinade is half that found in store-bought versions, and the fat comes from nutrient rich extra-virgin olive oil.

Ingredients

⅓ cup white vinegar

¼ cup extra-virgin olive oil

¼ cup freshly squeezed lemon juice

3 cloves garlic, peeled and minced

1 tablespoon dried parsley

1 tablespoon dried basil

½ teaspoon dried oregano

½ teaspoon garlic powder

½ teaspoon ground sea salt

½ teaspoon freshly ground black pepper

Directions

1. In a small mixing bowl or a salad dressing shaker, combine all the ingredients, and whisk or shake, mixing thoroughly.

Nutrition Facts (per serving)

70 calories, 7 grams fat, 1 gram saturated fat, 0 grams trans fat, 0 milligrams cholesterol, 135 milligrams sodium, 2 grams carbohydrates, 0 grams fiber, 0 grams sugar, 0 grams protein

HONEY VINAIGRETTE

Yield: 16 servings (1 tablespoon each)

Before:

One serving of typical store-bought salad dressing has 300 to 500 milligrams of sodium, which can quickly push you over your maximum daily sodium target.

Skinny-Size It:

Making your own salad dressing takes only a matter of minutes, and the bonus comes from controlling the amount of sugar in the dressing and skipping the salt all together. The salt will not even be missed, because of the flavorful spices that are added.

Ingredients

½ cup white vinegar

¼ cup canola oil

3 tablespoons honey

½ tablespoon Dijon mustard

1 teaspoon garlic powder

½ teaspoon freshly ground black pepper

Directions

1. In a small mixing bowl or a salad dressing shaker, combine all the ingredients, and whisk or shake, mixing thoroughly.

Nutrition Facts (per serving)

45 calories, 3.5 grams total fat, 0 grams saturated fat, 0 grams trans fat, 0 milligrams cholesterol, 0 milligrams sodium, 4 grams carbohydrates, 0 grams fiber, 3 grams sugar, 0 grams protein

GUILTLESS THOUSAND ISLAND DRESSING

Yield: 24 servings (1 tablespoon each)

Before:

Store-bought creamy salad dressings typically weigh in at around 60 calories per tablespoon and contain 5 grams of fat or more.

Skinny-Size It:

Making your own Guiltless Thousand Island Dressing requires only three simple ingredients, and a single serving has only 20 calories and 1.5 grams of fat.

Ingredients

1 cup reduced-fat mayonnaise

¼ cup ketchup

3 tablespoons sweet pickle relish

Directions

1. In a small bowl, combine all the ingredients, and mix well.
2. Store the dressing in an airtight container in the refrigerator for up to 7 days.

Nutrition Facts (per serving)

20 calories, 1.5 grams total fat, 0 grams saturated fat, 0 grams trans fat, 0 milligrams cholesterol, 135 milligrams sodium, 3 grams carbohydrates, 0 grams fiber, < 1 gram sugar, 0 grams protein

AVOCADO SALSA

Yield: 4 servings

Before:

In general, salsas are loaded with sodium from added salt. While tomato-based salsas tend to be fat free, adding in healthy fats, like monounsaturated fat from avocados, can be heart healthy and can slim the middle.

Skinny-Size It:

Lite soy sauce, hot sauce and wasabi are incorporated into this salsa to kick up the flavor, resulting in only 150 milligrams of sodium per serving. And each serving of this salsa has 8 grams of monounsaturated fat from the avocados and 6 grams of fiber. It is delicious served with multigrain tortilla chips or sliced fresh vegetables and is a perfect topping for many dishes.

Skinny Skip:

When preparing recipes, especially sauces, you can often skip or skimp on the salt, instantly reducing the amount of added sodium. If you must add salt to a dish, do so after serving and don't stir it in. This will allow the salt sprinkled over the food to hit your taste buds and quench your desire for salt.

Ingredients

2 medium ripe Hass avocados, halved, pit removed and peeled

½ small red onion, peeled and minced

2 medium scallions, root ends removed and finely diced

Juice of 3 limes (about 6 tablespoons)

2 teaspoons lite soy sauce

1 teaspoon prepared wasabi (green horseradish)

¼ teaspoon hot sauce

Directions

1. Place the avocado halves in a medium mixing bowl, and mash them with a fork, leaving small chunks.
2. Add the remaining ingredients and stir until just combined. Serve at once.

Nutrition Facts (per serving)

160 calories, 13 grams fat, 2 grams saturated fat, 0 grams trans fat, 0 milligrams cholesterol, 150 milligrams sodium, 12 grams carbohydrates, 6 grams fiber, 2 grams sugar, 2 grams protein

CREAMY BALSAMIC DRESSING

Yield: 24 servings (1 tablespoon each)

Before:

Salad dressings get their creaminess from cheese and cream.

Skinny Shopping:

Agave nectar is worth having on hand as it has a more intense sweetness and flavor than traditional granulated sugar. However, this doesn't mean that you should go crazy with agave nectar, as it is still a source of sugar and overall intake needs to be limited.

Skinny-Size It:

This dressing has a cream base from whipped cashews, which adds excellent flavor to the dressing. Then perk up the dressing with balsamic vinegar, garlic powder and agave nectar, for a little sweetness. The result is a dressing with 0 milligrams of sodium per serving. Last but not least, even with the healthiest of dressings, keep the serving size to 1 tablespoon!

Ingredients

1 cup raw cashews

1½ cups water, plus ¼ cup water for blending

1 tablespoon agave nectar

¼ cup balsamic vinegar

1 teaspoon garlic powder

Directions

1. Soak the cashews in the 1½ cups of water in a medium-size bowl, cover and refrigerate overnight to soften the nuts.

2. Drain the cashews and place them in a food processor or a blender along with the agave nectar, the vinegar, the remaining ¼ cup water and the garlic powder. Blend until smooth.

3. Store the dressing in an airtight container in the refrigerator for up to 7 days. If needed, thin the dressing by adding a teaspoon of water at a time.

Nutrition Facts (per serving)

30 calories, 2 grams total fat, 0 grams saturated fat, 0 grams trans fat, 0 milligrams cholesterol, 0 milligrams sodium, 2 grams carbohydrates, 0 grams fiber, 1 gram sugar, < 1 gram protein

GARLIC TOMATO SPAGHETTI SAUCE

Yield: 8 servings (½ cup each)

Before:

Store-bought spaghetti sauces typically have about 400 milligrams of sodium in each serving.

Skinny-Size It:

If you incorporate lots of fresh vegetables and garlic into your spaghetti sauce, you won't even miss the salt. This recipe has only 150 milligrams of sodium per serving. The Applesauce (see recipe on page 149), an unexpected addition, lends a light, natural sweetness to the sauce and helps thicken it. As the sauce simmers, all the flavors come together. Garlic Tomato Spaghetti Sauce is perfect for any dish calling for spaghetti sauce, from spaghetti squash and whole-wheat pasta to lasagna and eggplant Parmesan.

Skinny Shopping:

Look for elephant garlic. As the name suggests, its cloves are huge, making chopping them a breeze. Although the giant cloves will not fit in a garlic press, they are super easy to peel. Peeling regular-size cloves is a breeze if you use a garlic press. Place 1 or 2 cloves in a garlic press and squeeze gently. The peel will detach from the clove.

Ingredients

1 tablespoon extra-virgin olive oil

1 medium sweet onion, peeled and diced
(about 1 cup)

1 medium zucchini, ends cut off and diced (about 1 cup)

½ large red bell pepper, seeded, deribbed and diced
(about 1 cup)

2 teaspoons minced garlic

3 cups canned whole tomatoes (with juice)

One 15-ounce can diced tomatoes

½ cup Applesauce (see recipe on page 149)

1 teaspoon garlic powder

Directions

1. Heat the olive oil in a large pot over medium heat.
    Add the onions, zucchini, peppers and minced garlic
    and sauté for 5 to 7 minutes, or until the vegetables
    are tender.
2. Add the whole tomatoes, diced tomatoes, Applesauce
    and garlic powder, and bring to a boil. Then lower the
    heat to low and simmer for 45 minutes.
3. Store the spaghetti sauce in an airtight container in
    the refrigerator for up to 7 days.

Nutrition Facts (per serving)

70 calories, 2 grams total fat, 0 grams saturated fat, 0 grams trans
fat, 0 milligrams cholesterol, 150 milligrams sodium, 10 grams
carbohydrates, 2 grams fiber, 6 grams sugar, 2 grams protein

YOGURT TZATZIKI

Yield: 16 servings (2 cups in all)

Before:

Many creamy dips derive their flavor from added salt and have 100 calories or more per serving. Nearly all the calories come from fat, which can quickly undermine the nutritional value of the healthy foods served with these dips.

Skinny-Size It:

This yogurt-based tzatziki has only 10 calories per serving and gets its flavor from fresh herbs and cucumbers. It's very versatile, as it makes an excellent salad dressing and vegetable dip, and it even goes well with grilled chicken.

Ingredients

1 cup plain nonfat Greek yogurt

1 medium cucumber, grated (about 1 cup)

2 tablespoons minced fresh mint

2 tablespoons minced fresh dill

1 tablespoon freshly squeezed lemon juice

$\frac{1}{2}$ teaspoon sea salt

Directions

1. In a small mixing bowl, combine all the ingredients, and mix well.

2. Store the tzatziki in an airtight container in the refrigerator for up to 7 days.

Nutrition Facts (per serving)

10 calories, 0 grams fat, 0 grams saturated fat, 0 grams trans fat, 0 milligrams cholesterol, 80 milligrams sodium, 1 gram carbohydrates, 0 grams fiber, < 1 gram sugar, 2 grams protein

7
....

Drinks and Smoothies

Drinks such as iced tea, cocktails, lemonade and smoothies can wind up being loaded with sugar and can contribute basically empty calories, which have little to no nutritional value. By including fruits and vegetables in each recipe, these otherwise super-sugary drinks are transformed into versions that you want to get hooked on.

To stay true to Skinny Rule #6, "Skip the Soft Drinks— *Even Diet,*" these drinks are lower in calories and sugar without turning to sugar substitutes and diet mixers. The goal is to skimp on sugar. In my opinion, cutting back on the quantity of real sugar is better than swapping sugar for calorie-free sugar substitutes. Plus, incorporating fresh fruits and vegetables is an excellent way to add sweetness without scooping in piles of sugar. As you make these Skinny-Size It drinks and smoothies, I will toast to you. Here's to your health!

STRAWBERRY *MOJITO*

Yield: 2 servings

Before:

Most *mojito* recipes have more calories than you may think, and most of the calories come from sugar! Many *mojito* recipes call for 2 tablespoons of simple syrup (aka sugar) per cocktail. Plus, many restaurants make *mojitos* with tonic water, which adds about another 5 to 6 teaspoons of sugar per cocktail.

Skinny-Size It:

Eliminating the simple syrup in this drink and incorporating fresh strawberries lightens up the calories and, of course, slashes the sugar count to only 2 grams per serving, while still delivering a refreshing cocktail.

Skinny Tip:

Skip the rum and this recipe quickly becomes Skinny Strawberry Lime Water. You can keep a pitcher of this in the refrigerator for a refreshing summer drink with only 20 calories per glass. It's really thirst quenching when served over ice.

Ingredients

1 lime, sliced into 6 wedges

8 fresh mint leaves, plus 2 mint sprigs for garnishing

4 strawberries, stems removed and cut in half,
   plus 2 whole strawberries for garnishing

2 ounces white rum

Club soda

Ice

Directions

1. Place 3 lime wedges and 4 mint leaves in each of 2
    glasses and lightly mash in the bottom of the glass with
    a spoon or wooden muddler. Then add 2 strawberries
    to each glass and lightly muddle.
2. Top each glass with rum, club soda and ice. Garnish each
    with a strawberry and a sprig of mint, and serve at once.

Nutrition Facts (per serving)

80 calories, 0 grams fat, 0 grams saturated fat, 0 grams trans fat,
0 milligrams cholesterol, 0 milligrams sodium, 6 grams carbohydrates, 2 grams fiber, 2 grams sugar, < 1 gram protein

MOCHA FREEZE

Yield: 1 serving

Before:

At a coffee shop a frozen mocha coffee drink could have
about 400 calories and upwards of 16 grams of fat and
60 grams of sugar. While some of the sugar is naturally
occurring milk sugar, the majority is added sugar.

Skinny-Size It:

Thanks to frozen dark chocolate almond milk, this refreshing drink has only 120 calories per serving and about a third of the sugar compared to the coffee shop version.

Ingredients

1 cup dark chocolate almond milk (such as Silk), frozen in an ice cube tray

1 cup brewed coffee, iced

Directions

1. In a blender, combine the frozen almond milk cubes and coffee. Blend until smooth. Serve at once.

Nutrition Facts (per serving)

120 calories, 2.5 grams fat, 0 grams saturated fat, 0 grams trans fat, 0 milligrams cholesterol, 190 milligrams sodium, 23 grams carbohydrates, 1 gram fiber, 21 grams sugar, 2 grams protein

CHOCOLATE CHIA DRINK

Yield: 1 serving

This is a drink recipe that my sister introduced me to!

Before:

Most chocolate milk does not have fiber or omega-3 fatty acids in it.

Skinny-Size It:

Mixing up your own chocolate milk with chia seeds is a great way to add heart-helping omega-3 fatty acids and fiber to your diet. Each serving of Chocolate Chia Drink contains 1 gram of omega-3 fatty acids and 3 grams of fiber. An added bonus is that chia seeds are hydrophilic, holding ten times their weight in water, which means that this drink will fill you up naturally.

Ingredients

1 cup dark chocolate almond milk (such as Silk)

1 teaspoon chia seeds

1 teaspoon (or less) sugar (optional)

Directions

1. Pour the almond milk in a glass and then stir in the chia seeds. If you find the drink needs a little more sweetness, add sugar.

Nutrition Facts (per serving)

140 calories, 4 grams fat, 0 grams saturated fat, 0 grams trans fat, 0 milligrams cholesterol, 190 milligrams sodium, 25 grams carbohydrates, 3 grams fiber, 21 grams sugar, 3 grams protein

GREEN SMOOTHIE

Yield: 3 servings (1 cup each)

Before:

Smoothies are typically full of carbohydrates, have added sugar but lack healthy fats.

Skinny-Size It:

Adding avocado to a smoothie adds creaminess and mono-unsaturated fat, which is linked to reduced belly fat. A single serving of this smoothie provides 3 grams of monounsaturated fat. The Green Smoothie derives its natural sweetness from a blend of pineapple and mango, doing away with the need for any added sweetener. Additionally, the blend of greens and fruit in a serving provides 45 percent of the daily value for vitamin A and 100 percent of the daily value for vitamin C.

Skinny Shopping:

Stock up on frozen fruit, such as mango and berries, as they are perfect additions to smoothies and other recipes and taste great thawed. Opt for varieties that are plain and have no added sugar.

Ingredients

2 cups baby spinach

10 ounces fresh pineapple, cut into chunks

½ medium ripe Hass avocado, peeled

½ cup frozen mango chunks

½ cup low-fat vanilla yogurt or almond milk yogurt

¼ cup mango or orange juice

Directions

1. In a blender, combine all the ingredients and blend until smooth. Serve at once.

Nutrition Facts (per serving)

160 calories, 4.5 grams fat, 0.5 grams saturated fat, 0 grams trans fat, 0 milligrams cholesterol, 45 milligrams sodium, 26 grams carbohydrates, 4 grams fiber, 19 grams sugar, 6 grams protein

BANANA-PEACH SMOOTHIE

Yield: 2 servings

Before:

Most low-fat smoothies from restaurants use yogurt that has added sugar and syrups for flavoring. Some of these smoothies have as much as 48 grams of sugar per serving—with about three-quarters of the calories in the smoothie coming directly from the sugar.

Skinny Tip:

Frozen bananas are great in smoothies—buy a bunch of ripe bananas, remove the peels, place them in a freezer bag and freeze them to use later in smoothies.

Skinny-Size It:

To rein in the sugar, use plain nonfat Greek yogurt in your smoothie and sweeten it with fresh fruit, some 100 percent fruit juice and a little bit of honey or agave nectar. Using frozen fruit results in a smoothie that is icy, smooth and thick.

In addition to having much less sugar than conventional smoothies, the Banana–Peach Smoothie boasts 2 grams of fiber and 13 grams of protein per serving to fill you up!

Ingredients

1 cup plain nonfat Greek yogurt

1 cup frozen sliced peaches (no juice or sugar added)

1 medium frozen banana

¼ cup 100 percent orange juice

1 tablespoon honey or agave nectar

Directions

1. In a blender, combine all the ingredients and blend until smooth. Serve at once.

Nutrition Facts (per serving)

180 calories, 0 grams fat, 0 grams saturated fat, 0 grams trans fat, 0 milligrams cholesterol, 55 milligrams sodium, 34 grams carbohydrates, 2 grams fiber, 28 grams sugar, 13 grams protein

MANGO-COCONUT SMOOTHIE

Yield: 2 servings

Before:

If you look at the ingredients list for some fruit-flavored smoothies, you may not even see fruit listed, as sugary syrups are oftentimes used to add flavor instead of fruit.

Skinny-Size It:

This smoothie has frozen mango for flavor and sweetness, plain nonfat Greek yogurt for creaminess and coconut oil for a tropical flavor boost. While the coconut oil adds saturated fat to the smoothie, new research shows that not all types of saturated fat are created equal. For example, saturated fat from plant-based foods (such as coconut oil) has about 7 grams of lauric acid—a medium-chained saturated fat that, according to the latest science, does no harm to health. Plus coconut oil is potentially linked to decreasing inflammation and improving healthy (HDL) cholesterol levels.

Skinny Shopping:

Coconut oil is available in grocery stores and is typically found near other oils in the natural food section of the store.

Ingredients

1 cup frozen mango

1 cup plain nonfat Greek yogurt

¼ cup 100 percent orange juice

1 tablespoon honey

1 tablespoon coconut oil

Directions

1. In a blender, combine all the ingredients and blend until smooth. Serve at once.

Nutrition Facts (per serving)

230 calories, 7 grams fat, 6 grams saturated fat, 0 grams trans fat, 0 milligrams cholesterol, 55 milligrams sodium, 31 grams carbohydrates, 2 grams fiber, 28 grams sugar, 13 grams protein

PEACH-GINGER ICED TEA

Yield: 4 servings

Before:

Store-bought sweetened iced teas may look innocent, but some 16-ounce bottles contain 10 teaspoons' (40 grams) worth of added sugar or more! Typically, the sugar is pure sugar, not the sugar found in real fruit or fruit juice—even if there are images of fruit on the packaging.

Skinny-Size It:

Making your own flavored iced teas is a breeze. Using whole fruit instead of loading up on granulated sugar is the best way to tame the sugar. The sugar content of a serving of Peach-Ginger Iced Tea is just 4 grams, coming from fruit. Even if you added a teaspoon of sugar, you would still be way ahead of the game, compared to picking up bottled sweetened iced tea.

Skinny Shopping:

Stock up on a variety of flavored tea bags. Tea is great served iced or hot, and the calorie count is zero!

Ingredients

2 quarts hot water

4 peach-ginger tea bags (such as The Republic of Tea Ginger Peach Black or White Tea)

½ cup fresh or frozen peaches, cut into 1-inch pieces

Ice

½ fresh peach, cut into 4 slices, for garnish

Directions

1. Fill a large pitcher (one that is a little larger than 2 quarts) with the hot water and tea bags. Brew the tea for 15 minutes and then remove the tea bags. Add the peach chunks. Let the tea cool and then chill it in the refrigerator.

2. Serve the chilled tea over ice and garnish each glass with a fresh peach slice.

Nutrition Facts (per serving)

20 calories, 0 grams fat, 0 grams saturated fat, 0 grams trans fat, 0 milligrams cholesterol, 10 milligrams sodium, 4 grams carbohydrates, < 1 gram fiber, 4 grams sugar, 0 grams protein

SKINNY LEMONADE

Yield: 8 servings (8 ounces each)

Before:

Typical store-bought lemonade has about 11 or more teaspoons of sugar (about 46 grams) per 16-ounce serving, making this a drink you want to avoid.

Skinny-Size It:

Making your own lemonade requires only four ingredients: water, lemon juice, fresh lemon slices and sugar. I suggest using regular granulated sugar and just scaling back the amount that is added, although if you wish, you can use a sugar substitute instead. By kicking up the lemon flavor with the addition of fresh lemon slices, you won't even miss the sugar left out. With only 13 grams of sugar, Skinny Lemonade has just a fraction of the sugar found in conventional lemonade!

Skinny Swap:

You can reduce the sugar content of your lemonade even more by making one of my favorite drinks, the Arnold Palmer. It's simple! In a glass combine one part unsweetened iced tea and one part lemonade. That's it!

Ingredients

½ cup sugar

2 cups warm water, plus cold water for filling the pitcher

1 cup freshly squeezed lemon juice

1 medium lemon, seeded and sliced

Directions

1. Pour the sugar into a 2-quart pitcher and then add 2 cups warm water. Stir until the sugar has dissolved.
2. Add the lemon juice and lemon slices, and then fill the pitcher almost to the top with cold water. Chill the lemonade in the refrigerator and serve.

Nutrition Facts (per serving)

60 calories, 0 grams fat, 0 grams saturated fat, 0 grams trans fat, 0 milligrams cholesterol, 15 milligrams sodium, 16 grams carbohydrates, < 1 gram fiber, 13 grams sugar, 0 grams protein

TRIPLE BERRY OMEGA SMOOTHIE

Yield: 4 servings

Before:

Even the healthiest of smoothies tend to lack heart-helping omega-3 fatty acids.

Skinny Shopping:

Look in the refrigerated health food section of your grocery store or natural food store for Barlean's Pomegranate Blueberry Total Omega Swirl—it is a great staple to keep on hand. If you can't find it in a store, you can order it online from www.Barleans.com. Also, keep ice pop makers on hand, so that when you have leftover smoothie, you can freeze it as ice pops to enjoy later!

Skinny-Size It:

Use plenty of frozen fruit in your smoothie, and then boost the flavor and health benefits by adding a flavored omega oil, such as Barlean's Pomegranate Blueberry Total Omega Swirl. A single tablespoon has 1,623 milligrams (1.6 grams) of heart-helping omega-3 fatty acids. Thanks to the mixed berries, each serving of this Triple Berry Omega Smoothie has 80 percent of the daily value for immune-boosting vitamin C. This smoothie has such a great taste that I have to tell our sons, ages four and six, when they are clamoring for more that they have had all the fish oil they can have for the day—because as with most things in life, some is good for you, but more is not better. In fact, if you are taking fish oil supplements, skip them on the days you drink this smoothie. And when adapting recipes, use the amount of omega oil called for, because too much can have a blood-thinning effect in the body.

Ingredients

3 cups frozen mixed berries (no juice added)

1 cup plain nonfat Greek yogurt

¼ cup low-fat milk or almond milk

2 tablespoons Barlean's Pomegranate Blueberry Total Omega Swirl

Directions

1. In a blender, combine all the ingredients and blend until smooth. Serve at once.

Nutrition Facts (per serving)

130 calories, 3 grams fat, 0 grams saturated fat, 0 grams trans fat, 0 milligrams cholesterol, 35 milligrams sodium, 21 grams carbohydrates, 4 grams fiber, 12 grams sugar, 8 grams protein

CHOC-PB BANANA SHAKE

Yield: 2 servings

Before:

Restaurant chocolate shakes will not show up on any Skinny list! They can have a whopping 500-plus calories, 15 grams of fat or more and 100 grams of carbohydrates or more.

Skinny-Size It:

A Skinny shake made with dark chocolate almond milk, bananas and a little peanut butter is the perfect way to keep the calories, fat and carbs in check. The Choc-PB Banana Shake has only 240 calories, 7 grams of fat and 43 grams of carbohydrates per serving. Plus, it has all the sweetness a shake needs; just the right texture, thanks to the frozen bananas; and a boost of creaminess, healthy fat and protein, courtesy of the natural peanut butter. The end result is half the calories and fat compared to many conventional restaurant shakes, and the shake is so delicious, you won't even miss the other 250 calories.

Skinny Shopping:

Where you find almond milk varies from store to store. You may find it in a refrigerated cooler in the health food section of the store, or it may be in the dairy aisle, by the milk products, even though it is dairy free. Check, too, for shelf-stable 8-ounce boxes of almond milk, in case you'd rather not buy a half-gallon container. But almond milk is so delicious even by itself, a half gallon would likely not go to waste!

Ingredients

2 cups dark chocolate almond milk (such as Silk)

2 medium frozen bananas

1 tablespoon creamy natural peanut butter

Directions

1. In a blender, combine all the ingredients and blend until smooth. Serve at once.

Nutrition Facts (per serving)

240 calories, 7 grams fat, 0.5 grams saturated fat, 0 grams trans fat, 0 milligrams cholesterol, 189 milligrams sodium, 43 grams carbohydrates, 4 grams fiber, 31 grams sugar, 5 grams protein

CUCUMBER-MINT WATER

Yield: 8 servings

This recipe is for my aunts! There was a request to add some flavored water to *Skinny-Size It*. Perking up water by adding fresh flavor is super simple to do. I was introduced to cucumber water at a spa. It's refreshing, and with some added mint, it is extra refreshing!

Ingredients

8 cups cold water

½ cup thinly sliced cucumbers (with the peel), plus cucumber slices for garnishing

2 tablespoons minced fresh mint

Ice

Directions

1. Combine the water, cucumbers and mint in a 2-quart pitcher.
2. Pour in a glass over ice, garnish with a cucumber slice, and serve.

Nutrition Facts (per serving)

0 calories, 0 grams fat, 0 grams saturated fat, 0 grams trans fat, 0 milligrams cholesterol, 0 milligrams sodium, 0 grams carbohydrates, 0 grams fiber, 0 grams sugar, 0 grams protein

SKINNY GIN FIZZ

Yield: 2 servings

Before:

A traditional gin and tonic made with 8 ounces of tonic water has roughly 160 calories and 23 grams (almost 6 teaspoons) of sugar. All the sugar comes from the tonic water.

Skinny-Size It:

Bid farewell to tonic water and use naturally calorie-free, sugar-free club soda, which is the perfect base for a Skinny gin and tonic–like drink! Of course, garnish with plenty of lime slices to add refreshing flavor.

Ingredients

Ice

3 cups club soda

2 ounces gin

1 lime, cut into wedges or slices

Directions

1. Fill 2 glasses with ice, pour the club soda and gin over the ice, garnish with lime wedges or slices, and serve.

Nutrition Facts (per serving)

80 calories, 0 grams fat, 0 grams saturated fat, 0 grams trans fat, 0 milligrams cholesterol, 100 milligrams sodium, 2 grams carbohydrates, 0 grams fiber, 0 grams sugar, 0 grams protein

Skinny References

INTRODUCTION

Calorie Burn Calculator. Accessed May 10, 2013.
http://www.healthstatus.com

Reuters. "Eating in Restaurants Is Tied to Higher Calorie
Intake." Accessed May 10, 2013. http://www.reuters.com

The Salt (NPR blog). "Restaurant Meals Mean More Soda
for Kids." Accessed May 10, 2013. http://www.npr.org/blogs/
thesalt/

Stocking Your Skinny Kitchen

HHS and USDA. *Dietary Guidelines for Americans* (2010).
Accessed April 12, 2013. http://www.nlm.nih.gov/

"Sea Salt Vs. Table Salt." Accessed August 19, 2013.
http://www.heart.org

"Sodium in the Diet." Accessed April 20, 2013.
http://www.nlm.nih.gov/

"Lowering Salt in Your Diet." Accessed August 21, 2013.
http://www.fda.gov

WebMD. "The Truth about Agave." Accessed April 18, 2013. http://www.webmd.com

Skinny Tools

OXO Garlic Press. Accessed May 10, 2013. http://www.oxo.com

Tupperware Quick Shake Container. Accessed May 10, 2013. http://www.tupperware.com

Cuisinart 5-Cup Food Processor. Accessed May 10, 2013. http://www.cuisinart.com

Black & Decker 1½-Cup Food Chopper. Accessed May 10, 2013. http://www.amazon.com

Lodge Cast Iron Skillet. Accessed August 21, 2013. http://www.target.com

All-Clad Stainless-Steel Skillet. Accessed May 10, 2013. http://www.all-clad.com

Bamix Immersion Blender. Accessed May 10, 2013. http://www.bamix.com

Microplane Cut-Resistant Gloves. Accessed May 10, 2013. http://us.microplane.com

OXO Salad Spinner. Accessed May 10, 2013. http://www.oxo.com

Mini Colander. Accessed May 10, 2013. http://www.crateandbarrel.com

Calphalon 13-Inch Stainless Wok. Accessed May 10, 2013. http://www.calphalon.com

Oster Rice Cooker and Food Steamer. Accessed May 10, 2013. http://www.oster.com

Skinny Skimps, Swaps and Skips

Ener-G Egg Replacer. Accessed April 6, 2013.
http://www.ener-g.com

1 SKINNY-SIZE IT BREAKFAST

Ball, K., et al., "Socioeconomic Status and Weight Change in Adults: A Review." *Social Science & Medicine* 60 (2005): 1987–2010.

Keim, N. L., et al., "Weight Loss is Greater with Consumption of Large Morning Meals and Fat-Free Mass is Preserved with Large Evening Meals in Women on a Controlled Weight Reduction Regimen." *Journal of Nutrition* 127 (1997): 75–82.

Purslow, L. R., et al., "Energy Intake at Breakfast and Weight Change: Prospective Study of 6,764 Middle-aged Men and Women." *American Journal of Epidemiology* 167 (2008): 188–92.

Oatmeal Omega Parfait

Definition of *steel-cut oats.* Accessed April 16, 2013.
http://www.food.com

Tropical Mango Oatmeal

Eat + Run (*U.S. News & World Report* blog). "Dietary Fat: The Good, the Bad and the Ugly." Accessed March 18, 2013. http://health.usnews.com/health-news/blogs/eat-run/

2 SANDWICHES, SALADS AND SOUPS

Nutrition Facts for Taco Salad. Accessed May 10, 2013. http://www.tacobell.com

Avocado Reubens

Nutrition Facts for Reuben Sandwich. Accessed May 1, 2013. http://www.fitday.com

BBQ Tempeh Sandwich

Meatless Monday. Accessed March 24, 2013. http://www.meatlessmonday.com

Nutrition Facts for Lightlife Organic Three Grain Tempeh. Accessed May 4, 2013. http://www.lightlife.com

Mixed-Up Cobb Salad

Nutrition Facts for Cobb Salad. Accessed April 29, 2013. http://www.myfitnesspal.com

Veggie Chili

"Reducing Sodium in Canned Beans." Accessed September 23, 2013. http://www.todaysdietitian.com

French Onion Soup

French Onion Soup Nutrition Facts. Accessed April 29, 2013. http://www.myfitnesspal.com

3 HEALTHY ENTRÉES

"Choose My Plate." Accessed May 4, 2013.
  http://www.choosemyplate.gov

"How Size and Color of Plates and Tablecloths Trick Us
  Into Eating Too Much." Accessed May 7, 2013.
  http://www.forbes.com

Blackened Salmon with Mango Salsa

"Taking Omega-3 Supplements May Help Prevent Skin
  Cancer, New Study Finds." *Science Daily.* Accessed March
  18, 2013. http://www.sciencedaily.com/

"Seafood Dos and Don'ts When Pregnant." Accessed
  August 19, 2013. http://www.eatright.org

Traditional General Tso's Chicken

History of General Tso's Chicken. Accessed May 9, 2013.
  http://appetiteforchina.com

Polenta Lasagna

Nutrition Facts for Lasagna. Accessed May 9, 2013.
  http://www.olivegarden.com

4 DELICIOUSLY SKINNY SIDES

"Choose My Plate." Accessed March 20, 2013.
  http://www.choosemyplate.gov

Wansink, B., et al., "Super Bowls: Serving Bowl Size and
  Food Consumption." *JAMA* 230 (2005): 1727–28.

Sweet Potato Fries

Nutrition Facts for Sweet Potato Fries. Accessed May 6, 2013. http://www.myfitnesspal.com

5 SNACKS AND APPETIZERS

Potato Skinnies

Nutrition Facts for Potato Skins. Accessed April 23, 2013. http://www.tgifridays.com

PB Pretzel Granola

Nutrition Facts for Peanut Butter Pretzel Bar. Accessed May 6, 2013. http://www.clifbar.com

6 SAUCES, DRESSINGS AND DIPS

Skinny-Size It Hummus

Nutrition Facts for Hummus. Accessed May 7, 2013. http://www.athenos.com

Honey-Sesame Soy Sauce

Nutrition Facts for Asian Sauce. Accessed April 24, 2013. http://www.caloriecount.com

Maple BBQ Sauce

Nutrition Facts for Barbecue Sauce. Accessed April 25, 2013. http://www.caloriecount.com

7 DRINKS AND SMOOTHIES

Chocolate Chia Drink

Definition of *hydrophilic*. Accessed May 6, 2013. http://www.biology-online.org

Mango-Coconut Smoothie

"Is All Saturated Fat the Same?" *Huffington Post*. Accessed April 20, 2013. http://www.huffingtonpost.com

"Once a Villain, Coconut Oil Charms the Health Food World." *The New York Times*. Accessed August 23, 2013. http://www.nytimes.com

Index

Index

Index

Index

Index

[2]